# Farm Animal Welfare

# FARM ANIMAL
# WELFARE

## Social, Bioethical, and Research Issues

## BERNARD E. ROLLIN

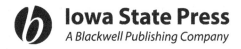

**Iowa State Press**
*A Blackwell Publishing Company*

**Bernard E. Rollin** is Professor of Philosophy, Professor of Physiology and Biophysics, and Director of Bioethical Planning at Colorado State University, Fort Collins. He is the author of more than 150 papers and ten books on animal welfare, genetic engineering, veterinary ethics, and bioethics.

© 1995 Iowa State University Press

Iowa State Press
A Blackwell Publishing Company
2121 State Avenue, Ames, Iowa 50014

Orders:       1-800-862-6657
Office:        1-515-292-0140
Fax:           1-515-292-3348
Web site:    www.iowastatepress.com

♾ Printed on acid-free paper in the United States of America

First edition, 1995
First paperback edition, 2003

The Library of Congress has cataloged the hardcover edition of this book as follows:

Rollin, Bernard E.
        Farm animal welfare: social, bioethical, and research issues/Bernard E. Rollin.—1st ed.
             p.            cm.
        Includes bibliographical references (p.       ) and index.
        ISBN 0-8138-2563-6 (acid-free paper)
        1. Livestock industry—Moral and ethical aspects. 2. Livestock—Research—Moral and ethical as-
pects. 3. Animal welfare. 4. Animal experimentation—Moral and ethical aspects. I. Title.
        HV4757.R65      1995
        179'.3—dc20                                                                              95-21992

Last digit is the print number:  9  8  7  6  5  4  3  2  1

TO MY FAMILY: **Linda, Mike, Yetta, Bob, Gwen, and Susie**

AND TO THE MEMORY OF **Peggy Jordan**

# Contents

# Preface

In 1980, writing in reference to the burgeoning social issue of the use, care, and treatment of animals in research, I pointed out that social debate on that topic was essentially little more than trench warfare, with each side lobbing mortar shells at the unseen, unheard other. Opponents of animal research demanded abolition; proponents demanded laissez-faire. It was clear to me that neither extreme would prevail and that meaningful answers to social concerns could be found only in the *via media*. In the attempt to find that middle way, a group of Colorado scientists and animal advocates drafted federal legislation that we believed would improve the lot of animals used in research while avoiding mindless bureaucratic hurdles to scientific activity. I articulated our approach in a book and was rewarded by a barrage of abuse from both extremes. A book review in a major medical journal called me an "apologist for the lab trashers," and an animal advocacy journal, not to be outdone, accused me of "selling out" and of "accepting the reality of science." Nonetheless, the legislation passed in 1985, and both sides now generally admit that it was the best that could be achieved. Few animal advocates would deny that it has significantly improved the life of research animals; few research advocates would claim that it has paralyzed research—indeed, many scientists believe it has made for better research by focusing attention on variables such as pain and distress which can skew results.

This example illustrates a conundrum about social change in our pluralistic, democratic society. First, such change invariably occurs in the middle: rarely do extremes prevail once an issue has reached public attention. At the same time, we tend to be contemptuous of advocates of middle positions, whom we view as "wimpy," "fence-straddling," "namby-pamby," and "lacking the courage of their convictions." Though we invariably end up in the middle, it is somehow unseemly to start there—it is as if we must first batter each other to a pulp. From a social perspective, perhaps it would be rational to seek the middle at the outset; it would certainly be more expeditious. I do not share the view that the middle is a place for cowards. Indeed, if we take the metaphor of the middle of the road literally, we remind ourselves that there is hardly a more dangerous place to stand than on the yellow line.

This book is an attempt to find the middle ground in the area of farm animal well-being. Society probably consumes more animals in agriculture than in all other areas combined; whereas the sum total of animals used in research numbers in the millions, the sum total of animals raised for food and fiber numbers in the billions. In addition, as the examples of Great Britain and Europe teach us, the welfare of farm animals is a paramount and growing concern to an increasingly urban populace and to many farmers as well. Animal agriculture thus involves a great many animal lives, a great deal of money, and a very high level of social concern. If we should ever be disposed to circumvent extremes and go directly to viable solutions, this is certainly the place. Yet here too we see trench warfare: animal advocates often demand an end to agriculture, and agribusiness proclaims that welfare is not an issue, that it is maximized in current production systems, and that everything is fine.

In the course of the discussion, I attempt to lay out in some detail the direction of the social consensus ethic vis-à-vis the treatment of farm animals, how this new ethic differs from traditional social ethics, and what can and should be done to accommodate the new ethical concerns. I examine each major agricultural use of animals, indicate its problematic dimensions pertaining to animal welfare, and suggest viable modifications and/or research to improve the situation. What is most surprising, I believe, is the significant extent to which answers to many of these problems already exist: what has most retarded progress in farm animal welfare is not the lack of answers but the failure to ask the questions.

In attempting this task, I fear I will once again be assaulted from both sides. Some animal advocates will castigate me for not attempting to abolish animal agriculture; some agriculturalists will see me, as one individual put it, as "a wolf in sheep's clothing." Nonetheless, I hope that most readers will see the wisdom of trying to do something meaningful and achievable to improve the current situation, as opposed to expending one's energy on quixotic crusades or on hurling invective.

I know from extensive personal experience that many scientists distance themselves from ethical issues, having been trained to believe that science is value-free and that ethical questions thus do not enter into the purview of scientific activity. This ideological perspective has caused significant mischief for both science and society in a variety of areas, including research on human subjects, animal research, and biotechnology, and has been a major force in eroding public confidence in science. If science is to contribute to the solution of social ethical issues, it must immerse itself in those issues, overcoming its ideological distance from such questions. I have explored this matter at length in *The Unheeded Cry: Animal Consciousness, Animal Pain, and Science* (Oxford University Press, 1989) and devote a significant amount of discussion in Part 1 of the present work to refuting elements of what I have called "the common sense of science," which serve as barriers to successful scientific involvement in farm animal welfare issues. Unlike many scientists, I argue that the very concept of "animal welfare" is inescapably and inextricably bound up with ethical notions.

In the end, animals cannot speak or advocate for themselves. Although that should inspire in us a sense of urgency about achieving progress regarding their well-being, the situation is often quite the opposite. In fact, we often soar to new heights of absurdity when we deal with animal issues, because animals, unlike disenfranchised human groups, cannot call us to account. If this book succeeds in helping to bring the discussion of farm animal welfare back down to earth, it will have accomplished its goal.

# Acknowledgments

The issue of farm animal welfare has great importance for agriculture, society, and government. Nonetheless, it is one which industry and government have traditionally failed to engage and about which society is largely uninformed. It is, furthermore, a multifaceted, multidisciplinary subject, combining matters of social ethics and philosophy, economics, agriculture, public perception, and science.

I am grateful to United States Department of Agriculture/Cooperative State Research Service for asking me to assay a rational approach to understanding—and dealing with—the complex cluster of questions embodied in the issue of farm animal welfare. In particular, I especially thank Dr. John Patrick Jordan, former CSRS administrator, for his vision, courage, moral commitment, and incisive criticisms.

I was greatly heartened by the response of the agricultural community to my undertaking this project. Early in my work, one member of the swine industry expressed the position I was to hear from diverse elements of agriculture: "This is very important; it must be done; and you are in a perfect position to do it, since you are as credible to both sides as anyone could be."

Without the help and support, moral and practical, I received from the agriculture and agricultural research communities, I could not have completed this project. I found many mentors: kind, open, patient, and possessed of the directness and honesty that is a hallmark of agricultural people and the agriculture ethic. These people include:

| | | |
|---|---|---|
| Jack Albright | Garth Boyd | Tom Field |
| Brad Anderson | Reeves Brown | Ted Friend |
| Jack Avens | Suzanne Dern | Frank Garry |
| Bill Baumgardt | Ian Duncan | Temple Grandin |
| Tim Blackwell | John Edwards | Glenn Gray |

| Mark Haake | Nathan Moreng | Ray Stricklin |
|---|---|---|
| Frank Hurnik | Bob Mortimer | Carolyn Struhl |
| Larue Johnson | Ken Odde | Steve Suther |
| Dawson Jordan | Bill O'Hare | Robert Taylor |
| Tony Knight | Edward Price | Gary Teague |
| Chris Losch | George Seidel | Jim Voss |
| Lonnie Losch | Gary Smith | Bill Wagner |
| Joy Mench | Joe Stookey | Bill Wailes |

I am also grateful to the thousands of farmers, ranchers, and other agriculturalists, including bankers, extension agents, and veterinarians, with whom I have discussed these issues for over fifteen years.

I have benefited much from dialogue with many people outside agriculture. They include:

| Adele Douglas | Dick Kitchener | Andrew Rowan |
|---|---|---|
| Mike Fox | Michael Losonsky | Steve Sapontzis |
| Terry Gipps | Jim Mason | Joyce Tischler |
| Gordon Glover | Linda Rollin | Tom Wolfle |
| Lynne Kesel | Mike Rollin | |

In preparing the manuscript, I had the invaluable help of Alicia Boscarelli, Hollye Gonzales, and Dennis Sylvan.

I am grateful to USDA/CSRS for funding the study out of which this book grew.

# The Social and Bioethical Background

Animal producers, animal scientists, and agriculturalists in general react in a paradoxical way to the emerging social/ethical concerns about the well-being of farm animals. On the one hand, critics of intensive agriculture are almost universally characterized as kooks and vegetarian extremists, or else as cynical opportunists. For example, a cartoon widely disseminated by the Animal Industry Foundation and captioned, "What do these folks know about animal agriculture?" depicts just such an array of individuals. (Unfortunately, the foundation did not allow me to reproduce the cartoon in this book.) The disreputable characters are recognizable as a dotty old woman in Birkenstocks; an illiterate punker; an opportunistic photojournalist; a wealthy, radical chic couple, complete with pampered poodle; an egghead academic; and an aging, burned-out hippie. Such stereotyping of "humaniacs" seems to reassure agriculturalists that they are dealing with a radical, extremist fringe phenomenon that has no serious content and is thus no threat.

On the other hand, and at the same time, the agricultural community is highly threatened by these social concerns. It often ranks animal welfare as one of the three major challenges confronting agriculture as the new century dawns, the others being environmental issues and food-safety concerns.

The conflict between these two stances is, of course, patent. If concerns about animal well-being are overwhelmingly radical, fringe issues, they represent little danger to agriculture; at most, they are a petty nuisance. And if they are a significant problem, they cannot be merely the purview of the radical fringe, or else they would not pose much of a threat to what is after all a major industry. The great majority of the public consumes animal products, and society in general is never, by definition, radical. This basic point was well understood by a Texas cowboy who, after hearing me articulate it in a speech, remarked that I was quite correct and pointed out that if the issue of farm animal well-being existed merely in the minds and pronouncements of a few extremists, "we could shoot the sons-a-bitches."

In less colorful terms, thinking individuals realize that truly extremist ideas, which garner no support from society in general, are not a threat to the established order. Nevertheless, extremely radical people can serve to articulate, in an exaggerated way, the germ of ideas whose time is coming in society in general—U.S. history has recently witnessed this phenomenon with regard to both feminist and civil rights issues. If an idea is truly marginal, it is best ignored, for it will inevitably perish from lack of nourishment. But conversely, if radicals are simply stridently and hyperbolically anticipating something that is developing in the zeitgeist of society at large, it behooves those in positions of authority to separate wheat from chaff and find the core of concern. This core can be dealt with proactively and rationally before it is indeed usurped by radicals with their own agenda and before the radical account of the issues becomes the only account available to society in general.

The issue of farm animal welfare is a genuine issue of concern to social ethics. In the discussion, I attempt to show that such concerns are first of all mainstream, with radical voices simply exaggerating and overstating what must be heard. (Of course, some agriculturalists and agricultural scientists have recognized this fact.) Second, I argue that far from being radical, the social concerns are ultimately highly conservative, attempting to preserve values that are as old as human-animal interaction and animal agriculture itself. Before I explain the new ethic for animals that I argue is emerging in society, however, it is necessary to delineate some fundamental aspects of the traditional social ethic that obtained for animals virtually since the dawn of civilization, in order to contrast it with the new ethic.

It is, of course, also important to realize that those in society most concerned about animal welfare often stereotype producers as uncaring, avaricious rednecks with no concern for the animals. We shall see in our subsequent discussion that such a view is equally misinformed and that this stereotype must also be corrected.

# 1
## The New Social Ethic for Animals

## Personal Ethics and Social Ethics

Before embarking on a discussion of the traditional moral status of animals in society, it is necessary to review some fundamental features of ethics, whose logical aspects are often misunderstood. A basic distinction which must be drawn between two very different senses of ethics, which I shall designate ethics$_1$ and ethics$_2$. Ethics$_1$ is the set of rules, principles, and beliefs about right and wrong, good and bad, justice and injustice, duty and obligation which governs people's behavior, or which they believe ought to govern their behavior. Ethics$_2$, on the other hand, is the study, critique, analysis, and criticism of ethics$_1$—and thus is a philosophical activity, in the sense that it examines the logic and coherence of fundamental concepts and beliefs. Ethics$_1$ is taught by teachers, churches, parents, peers, movies, and the media; ethics$_2$ is generally taught in philosophy classes.

Under ethics$_1$, social ethics must be distinguished from personal ethics. Too many people make the mistake, in their ethics$_2$ moments, of assuming that all ethics$_1$ is subjective, a matter of opinion and not fact, and thus not subject to rational discussion. Although it is true that one cannot do experiments or gather data to decide what is right and wrong, that does not mean that ethics is whim and caprice. Anyone who doubts this may contemplate the fate of an individual who robs a bank in front of witnesses and then attempts to argue before a court that, in *his* ethical opinion, bank robbery is acceptable if one needs the money.

In other words, just because ethics$_1$ is not validated by gathering facts or doing experiments does not mean it is a matter of opinion. In fact, relatively little ethics is left to one's personal opinion. Consensus rules about rightness and wrongness of actions that have an impact on others are articulated in clear social principles that are encoded in laws and policies. All public regulations, from keeping of pornographic bookstores out of school zones to laws against insider trading and murder, are examples of consensus ethical principles written large in policy. Those portions of ethics that are universally binding and socially objective I call the *social consensus ethic*. A moment's reflection reveals that, without such a consensus ethic on fundamental matters, we would have chaos and anarchy, and society would be impossible. Thus the social consensus ethic is universally binding on members of society and is not a matter of opinion.

Now the social consensus ethic does leave certain areas of behavior to the discretion of the individual, or more accurately, to his or her *personal ethic*. Such things as what one reads, what one theologically believes or does not believe, how much charity one gives and to what groups are left in our society to one's personal beliefs about right and wrong. But it should be stressed again that what society considers absolutely fundamental to daily life is objectified in the consensus ethic.

It is also important to realize that, as society evolves over time, certain areas of conduct may move from the concern of the social consensus ethic to the concern of the personal ethic, and vice versa. An example of something that has recently moved from the concern of the social ethic and law to the purview of individual ethical choice is sexual behavior. Where once laws constrained such activities as homosexual behavior, adultery, and cohabitation, they are now left to one's personal ethic in U.S. society and in other Western democracies.

On the other hand, matters that have historically been the domain of the personal ethic may be appropriated by the social ethic and made a matter of law. This situation often occurs when society feels that some important moral principles or considerations are being abridged or neglected in virtue of leaving the area in question to personal discretion. Thus hiring and firing one's employees or renting one's real property, once paradigmatic examples of what was left to individual morality, have increasingly become matters of law, for it was felt that people were violating fundamental notions of fairness by not hiring women or by failing to sell or rent to blacks and other minorities. As we shall see, something similar is emerging regarding the treatment of animals.

## Traditional Social Ethics and the Treatment of Animals

For as long as humans have domesticated animals and have articulated a social consensus ethic, it has included an ethic for the treatment of animals, albeit a very limited one. That traditional ethic has been an ethic forbidding *cruelty* to animals, that is, deliberate, sadistic, useless, unnecessary infliction of pain, suffering, and neglect on animals.[1] The Bible condemns such cruelty, as when it proscribes yoking an ox and ass together to pull a plow: given their unequal strength, the weaker animal would suffer needlessly. Similarly, it condemns muzzling an ox when it is threshing grain, for the animal would be unable to eat yet would be tantalized by the food. The rabbinic tradition interprets slaughter by cutting of the throat with a sharp razor as an injunction against unnecessary animal suffering, since exsanguination in and of itself is relatively pain-free.

Ancient writers in the Greek tradition similarly denounced animal cruelty, as did (and does) orthodox Catholic theology, as enunciated by Thomas Aquinas. In the latter tradition, cruelty is largely condemned on the grounds that those who are cruel to animals have a tendency to go on and abuse people, a thesis that has been confirmed by modern psychology, most dramatically, perhaps, in the case of recent serial killers, all of whom had early histories of animal abuse. Studies have also demonstrated a close connection between child abuse and animal abuse. In any case, all civilized societies have spoken against cruelty as the essence of their consensus social ethic regarding animal treatment. In the last few decades, however, in Europe, North America, Australia, and elsewhere, society has demanded that our consensus social ethic move beyond cruelty. Is this demand mere fashion or is there a rational basis for it?

To answer this question, one must articulate the difference between traditional animal use and what has occurred over the last fifty years. For essentially all of human history, the overwhelming reason for domesticating and keeping animals has been agricultural. The raison d'être for agriculture has been the use of animals and their products for food, fuel, or fiber, or as a source of power for locomotion, plowing, grinding, carrying, and so on. In terms of numbers, agriculture still uses far and away the largest number of animals of any human pursuit. Other areas of animal use, such as research and testing, were statistically negligible until well into the twentieth century. So it is fair to equate the preponderance of human animal use with agriculture through virtually all of human civilization.

By the same token, certain constitutive features of animal agriculture were essentially constant across space and time until the mid-twentieth century. Most significant for our purposes was the symbiotic nature of animal agriculture, what I call the "social contract" between humans and animals. Humans provided food, forage, protection against extremes of weather and predation, and, in essence, the opportunity for the animals to live lives for which they were maximally adapted—better lives than they would live if left to fend for themselves. The animals in turn provided food, toil, fiber, and power for humans. The situation was thus a win/win one, with both animals and humans better off in the relationship than they would have been outside it.

The key feature, then, of traditional agriculture was good husbandry. And the essence of good husbandry was keeping the animals under conditions to which their natures were biologically adapted, and augmenting these natural abilities by providing additional food, protection, care, or shelter from extremes of climate, predators, disease, drought, and so on, and by selectively breeding better survival traits into their natures. (The very term *husbandry* is highly significant; etymologically, it means "bonded to the house.") Thus traditional animal agriculture involves piggybacking, as it were, on the natures and abilities of animals. If the animals thrived, the producers thrived. The animals' interests were the producers' interests. Ethics and prudence were closely intertwined: the biblical injunction to rest the animals on the Sabbath expressed both concern for animals and prudence; exhausted animals would not reproduce, produce, or work as well as rested ones. Ethics and self-interest were organically united; to this day, extensive cattle ranchers in the American West, those people whose activities most closely approximate traditional agriculture, affirm that "we take care of the animals—and the animals take care of us," and it is axiomatic to ranch children that the animals are fed and watered before they themselves eat or rest.

In this amalgam of human interest and animal interest, ethics and prudence, the strongest possible sanction existed against harming the animals—harm to the animals was harm to the farmer. Any prolonged suffering inflicted on an animal by a producer, any systematic attempt to violate or work against the animals' natures would ultimately work just as much against the producers' interests as against the interests of the animals. Traditional agriculture, therefore, was primarily about putting square pegs in square holes, round pegs in round holes, with as little friction as possible. Any affronts to the animals' interests, such as knife castration or hot-iron branding, were of necessity short-lived, and systematic infliction of anything that routinely abraded the animals' biological natures was inconceivable.

This is not to say that traditional agriculture was a bed of roses for the animals. Since human control of nature was severely limited, animals suffered from famine, drought, disease, extremes of climate, and so on. But animal suffering *at human hands* was minimized by the symbiosis described above. The coincidence of ethics and self-interest was nearly perfect—anyone who deliberately hurt an animal, except for the most exigent reasons, was necessarily deviant. To be sure, this idealized picture was sometimes distorted by custom or misconception, as occurred (and still occurs) in rough handling of cattle or brutal training of horses, but wise husbandrymen knew that "gentling" was best. To this day, ranchers are reluctant to hire rodeo competitors as ranch hands, for they are too often guilty of "cowboying" the animals, being athletes interested in developing or exhibiting a skill, not husbandrymen.

If a nineteenth-century agriculturalist, let alone an ancient one, had dreamed of keeping thousands of chickens in one building, such a scheme would have been soon corrected by nature, for it would be a rapid path to ruin, bringing quick spread of animal disease, death, and financial disaster. Producers did well if and only if animals did well, and—this is critical—"did well" for the animal meant playing out its biological nature in an environment for which those powers had been selected by both natural and artificial selection.

Society, therefore, did not need laws mandating good husbandry for animals—that was dictated by self-interest and reinforced by the ancient ethic of care. If a person did not care about self-interest, he or she was unlikely to be persuaded by laws. Punishing bad husbandrymen was redundant, for they were effectively self-punishing. This, in turn, explains why the traditional social consensus ethic for the treatment of animals—the anticruelty ethic and, later, the laws expressing it—could be so minimal yet socially adequate. Normal people cared for their animals: failure to care for animals; failure to provide food, water, and shelter; or eagerness to inflict pain and suffering bespoke sadism or pathology that was irrational, deviant, and needed to be socially punished. To this day, a powerful aversion to animal cruelty—that is, willfully and uselessly harming an animal, or harming an animal for frivolous reasons—is ingrained in virtually all agriculturalists, especially those who come from an extensive background. Indeed, by extracting this powerful and universal ethical maxim from cattlemen, one can also quickly extract moral self-examination about rodeo, which, though culturally sanctified among ranchers, is nonetheless a source of moral discomfort to them when they are led to measure it by their own ethic.

In sum, society has had a very minimal consensus ethic for the treatment of animals—the prohibition of deliberate cruelty—largely because animal abuse was fundamentally inimical to what agriculturalists, the primary animal users, were trying to accomplish. Given the almost perfect coincidence of moral concern for animals and producer and social self-interest, it was redundant to write that ethic large, in Plato's phrase, in social morality, for it was already presupposed. Only deviant, sadistic, senseless abuse represented a moral affront, and thus only such behavior became the focal point of concern for the social ethic about animal treatment.

Thus, until recently, the only socially pervasive concept for criticizing or even discussing animal treatment was the concept of cruelty (and its partner, kindness). Humane societies were chartered to prevent cruelty—witness the name of the first U.S. humane society, the American Society for Prevention of Cruelty to Animals (ASPCA). Indeed, the logo of the ASPCA depicts its founder, Henry Bergh, staying the hand of a carter who is brutally beating his horse. And throughout their history, humane societies have concentrated on prosecuting and exposing deliberate cruelty, both individual and institutionalized, such as dog fighting and cockfighting.

The anticruelty ethic was codified in anticruelty laws, which stressed that their purview was sadistic or deviant behavior toward animals, not standard agricultural practices, which were in fact exempted from such laws. To be sure, these laws were quite flawed in their implementation; prosecutors, judges, and police tended to give them low priority, and thus their effect was limited.[2] But they were not perceived as *conceptually flawed* as long as the primary social concern was deviant behavior, not standard agricultural practice. The former was thankfully relatively rare, the latter was presumed to be self-correcting for reasons discussed above.

## The Inadequacy of the Traditional Ethic

Except in the opinion of a few isolated thinkers,[3] the anticruelty ethic (and the laws expressing it) were by and large considered adequate to the social concerns about animal treatment until the mid-twentieth century. At this time a series of significant social changes brought about inchoate but gradually more precise new social thought about animals.

The end of World War II witnessed the emergence of two major patterns with profound implications for the traditional social ethic for animals. The first occurred in the area of animal use in biomedical research.[4] From 1900 to 1920, the number of animals used in such research was both low and constant. After 1920 the growth rate increased somewhat and then precipitously increased during and especially directly after World War II, when large amounts of money were pumped into research and drug production. Such activity reached a peak in the 1960s.

The second pattern occurred in agriculture and grew out of the industrialization of animal agriculture. Between World War II and the mid-1970s, agricultural productivity—including animal products—increased dramatically. In the hundred years between 1820 and 1920, agricultural productivity doubled. After that, productivity continued to double in much shorter and ever-decreasing time periods. The next doubling took thirty years (between 1920 and 1950); the subsequent doubling took fifteen years (1950–65); the next one took only ten years (1965–75). As R. E. Taylor points out, the most dramatic change took place after World War II, when productivity increased more than fivefold in thirty years.[5] Fewer workers were producing far more food. Just before World War II, 24 percent of the U.S. population was involved in production agriculture;[6] today the figure is well under 2 percent (1.7 percent). Whereas in 1940 each farm worker supplied food for eleven persons in the general population, by 1990 each farm worker was supplying eighty persons. At the same time, the proportion of disposable income spent on food dropped significantly, from 30 percent in 1950 to 11.8 percent in 1990.[7]

There is thus no question that industrialized agriculture, including animal agriculture, is responsible for greatly increased productivity. It is equally clear that the husbandry associated with traditional agriculture has changed significantly as a result of industrialization. Symbolically, Departments of Animal Husbandry in universities in the United States have changed their names to Departments of Animal Science, thereby marking an essential feature of the trend.

For our purposes, several aspects of technological agriculture must be noted. In the first place, as just mentioned, the number of workers has declined significantly, yet the number of animals produced has increased. This has been possible because of mechanization, technological advancement, and the consequent capability of confining large numbers of animals in highly capitalized facilities. Of necessity, less attention is paid to individual animals. Second, technological innovations have allowed us to alter the environments in which animals are kept. Whereas in traditional agriculture animals had to be kept in environments for which they had evolved, we can now keep them in environments that are contrary to their natures but congenial to increased productivity. Battery cages for laying hens and gestation crates for sows provide examples of this point (discussed in detail in Part 2). The friction thus engendered is controlled by technology. For example, crowding of poultry would once have been impossible because of flock decimation by disease; now antibiotics and vaccines allow producers to avoid this self-destructive consequence.

A moment's reflection on the development of large-scale animal research and high-technology agriculture elucidates why these innovations have led to the demand for a new ethic for animals in society. In a nutshell, this new technology represents a radically different playing field of animal use from the one that characterized most of human history; in the modern world of agriculture and animal research, the traditional ethic grows increasingly less applicable.

A thought experiment makes this clear. Imagine a pie chart that represents all the suffering that animals experience at human hands today. What percentage of that suffering is a result of intentional cruelty of the sort condemned by the anticruelty ethic and laws? When I ask my audiences this question—whether scientists, agriculturalists, animal advocates, or members of the general public—I always get the same response: only a fraction of 1 percent. Few people have ever witnessed overt, intentional cruelty, which is thankfully rare.

On the other hand, people realize that biomedical and other scientific research, toxicological safety testing, uses of animals in teaching, pharmaceutical product extraction from animals, and so on all produce far more suffering than does overt cruelty. This suffering comes from creating disease, burns, trauma, fractures, and the like in animals in order to study them; producing pain, fear, learned helplessness, aggression, and other states for research; poisoning animals to study toxicity; and performing surgery on animals to develop new operative procedures. In addition, suffering is engendered by the housing of research animals. Indeed, a prominent member of the biomedical research community has argued that the discomfort and suffering that animals used in research experience by virtue of being housed under conditions that are convenient for us but inimical to their biological natures—for example, keeping rodents, which are nocturnal, burrowing creatures, in polycarbonate cages under artificial, full-time light—far exceed the suffering produced by invasive research protocols.[8]

Now it is clear that researchers are not intentionally cruel—they are motivated by plausible and decent intentions: to cure disease, advance knowledge, ensure product safety, augment their résumés. Nonetheless, they may inflict great amounts of suffering on the animals they use. (This is not, of course, to suggest that *all* animal research involves pain and suffering.) Furthermore, the traditional ethic of anticruelty and the laws expressing it had no vocabulary for labeling such suffering, since researchers were not maliciously intending to hurt the animals. Indeed, this is eloquently marked by the fact that the cruelty laws exempt animal use in science from their purview.

Those who first recognized this suffering as a concern (by and large the humane societies), lacking any vocabulary to describe it, often called researchers cruel, but such a description was clearly inadequate and served only to shut down dialogue between such concerned people and the research community. A new set of concepts beyond cruelty and kindness was needed to discuss the issues associated with burgeoning research animal use.

Precisely the same point is true regarding criticism of confinement, industrialized agriculture. As we shall see, society eventually became aware that new kinds of suffering were engendered by this sort of agriculture. Once again, producers could not be categorized as cruel, yet they were responsible for new types of animal suffering on at least three fronts:

1. Production diseases arise from the new ways the animals are produced. For example, liver abscesses in cattle are a function of certain animals' responses to the high-concentrate, low-roughage diet that characterizes feedlot production. (That is, of course, not the only cause of liver abscesses.) Although a certain percentage of the animals get sick and die, the overall economic efficiency of feedlots is maximized by the provision of such a diet.

2. The huge scale of industrialized agricultural operations—and the

small profit margin per animal—militates against the sort of individual attention that typified much of traditional agriculture. A case that speaks to this point was sent to me by a veterinarian for commentary in the column that I write for the *Canadian Veterinary Journal*:

> You (as a veterinarian) are called to a 500-sow farrow-to-finish swine operation to examine a problem with vaginal discharges in sows. There are three full-time employees and one manager overseeing approximately five thousand animals. As you examine several sows in the crated gestation unit, you notice one with a hind leg at an unusual angle and inquire about her status. You are told, "She broke her leg yesterday and she's due to farrow next week. We'll let her farrow in here and then we'll shoot her and foster off her pigs." *Is it ethically correct to leave the sow with a broken leg for one week while you await her farrowing?*[9]

Before commenting on the case, I spoke to the veterinarian who had experienced this incident, a swine practitioner. He explained that such operations run on tiny profit margins and minimal labor. Thus, even when he offered to splint the leg at cost, he was told that the operation could not afford the manpower entailed by separating this sow and caring for her! At this point, he said, he realized that confinement agriculture had gone too far. He had been brought up on a family hog farm, where the animals had names and were provided individual husbandry, and the injured animal would have been treated or, if not, euthanized immediately. "If it is not feasible to do this in a confinement operation," he said, "there is something wrong with confinement operations!"

It is important to note that not all confinement operations would treat the injured sow in this manner. The large, highly capitalized hog operations I visited assured me that they would euthanize any such injured animal immediately. It is generally the smaller operations, run on a shoestring, that fall prey to the sort of problem described. It is also important to note that highly extensive agriculture can also lead to suffering by virtue of neglect. In New Zealand, many sheep are unattended at lambing, and if climatic conditions are not ideal, animals can be lost. Thus extensive agriculture, in and of itself, does not ensure that good husbandry is practiced.

3. The final new source of suffering in industrialized agriculture results from physical and psychological deprivation for animals in confinement: lack of space, lack of companionship for social animals, inability to move freely, boredom, austerity of environments, and so on (discussed in detail in Part 2). Since the animals evolved for adaptation to extensive environments but are now placed in truncated environments, such deprivation is inevitable. This was not a problem in traditional, extensive agriculture.

These sources of suffering, like the ones in research, are again not captured by the vocabulary of cruelty, nor are they proscribed or even acknowledged by the laws of the anticruelty ethic. Furthermore, they typically do not arise under the traditional agriculture and ethic of husbandry. The development of large-scale uses of animals in science and the (roughly) contemporaneous rise of intensive agriculture engendered significant amounts of new suffering for animals which could not be conceptually encompassed or even discussed in terms of the traditional social ethic proscribing cruelty. At the same time, as public awareness of this suffering increased, the concern for its alleviation and mitigation grew exponentially. Thus the need for a new ethic and a new set of ethical concepts adequate to these technological innovations was created.

Let me stress again that I do not mean to suggest that all intensive confinement operations are the same; there are, of course, well-managed and poorly managed intensive operations just as there were well-managed and poorly managed extensive operations. My point is to indicate sources of animal suffering that tend to arise out of the nature of confinement agriculture, not simply out of bad management. That the sow in the case discussed above was not euthanized may be bad management; but both the economic push not to euthanize her and the tendency of sows to experience such leg problems, as well as the general lack of attention to individual animals, stem from the nature of confinement operations. As we shall see in Part 2, even beautifully managed confinement swine operations using gestation crates must lead to deprivation of exercise, social contact, and stimulation for the sows.

## The Rise of the New Ethic

The emergence of a new ethic in response to changes in agricultural and research uses of animals was facilitated by a variety of sociocultural factors.

### The Urbanization of Society

Along with the development of confinement agriculture came a significant movement of population from rural communities to urban and suburban areas. Inevitably, a loss of direct connection with the nature of agriculture was experienced by the vast majority of the population. Although, as discussed above, agriculture changed dramatically in the second half of the twentieth century, public understanding of these changes was at first minimal, and most of the population still schematized agriculture in terms of the small, extensive unit typified in "Old MacDonald's Farm."[10] This stereotypical agrarian ideal was perpetuated by multiple factors, not the least of which was agriculture's self-promotion, as in the Perdue Company's advertisement boasting of raising "happy chickens" under what were depicted as barnyard conditions. Public consciousness was therefore shocked by its encounter with the realities of confinement agriculture. This was most obvious in Great Britain, where Ruth Harrison's 1964 book, *Animal Machines,*[11] introduced the British public to industrialized agriculture, galvanizing social concern to such an extent that the British government was forced to appoint a royal commission, the Brambell Commission, to examine the issue and make recommendations.[12] At the same time, attempts to articulate new moral categories that went beyond cruelty were sparked in Britain, primarily by the growing awareness of confinement agriculture.[13]

The same sort of concern about the discord between the public agrarian ideal and the realities of confinement agriculture surfaced in Sweden in the late 1980s, prompted by a campaign led by children's author Astrid Lindgren, who was appalled by the facts of confinement. Her feelings struck a responsive chord in Swedish society, which in 1988 passed legislation that severely restricted confinement agriculture.[14] The Swedish case provides a concrete example of the new ethic applied to agriculture in the political arena.

Augmenting the persistence of the agrarian ideal in urbanized society was a new way of looking at animals. Once again, a thought experiment clarifies this point expeditiously. Imagine traveling back in time one hundred years and stopping people on the street in either an urban or a rural setting. Imagine further subjecting these people to a word-association test wherein they are asked to state the first word that comes into their minds when you utter a word. Thus, suppose you say *steam*; they might say *engine.* You then utter the word *animal.* The vast majority of people at that time would undoubtedly respond with *cow, horse, food, farm,* and so on. Were one to attempt this today, the response would be very different. People would certainly reply with *dog, cat, pet, friend.* Nearly all the pet-owning population sees these animals as members of the family. In other words, a primarily utilitarian view of animals has been superseded by a more personal and comradely view.

## Media Exploitation

This personal view of animals, coupled with a lack of daily dependence on, intercourse with, or knowledge of animals for most of the population, has made animals a source of endless fascination to the general public. Books, movies, newspapers, and television programs are quick to exploit this passion and to augment it with both accurate and inaccurate anthropomorphic accounts of animals that an uninformed public cannot critically assess.

That "animals sell papers," as one reporter told me, has been proved repeatedly. Thus media coverage of animals in themselves, and of human exploitation and abuse of animals, finds a perennially interested and responsive audience. Concern about the welfare of animals used in science, agriculture, and other areas has been fueled by extensive press coverage. It is generally agreed that media reports of the 1984 University of Pennsylvania atrocities against laboratory animals in baboon head-injury studies, as documented on videotape by the researchers themselves,[15] rapidly accelerated public concern about animals used in research and thereby ensured passage of the federal legislation we shall shortly discuss.[16]

## The Social Context

The period from the 1950s to the present witnessed the rise of an ethics of social concern about traditionally ignored and exploited groups such as racial minorities, native populations, women, the disabled, children, Third World peoples, the mentally ill, powerless humans used in research, and endangered species and ecosystems. Exploitation of any sort became suspect, and new generations were significantly sensitized to any kind of injustice or unfairness. Ecological consciousness stressed our kinship with other inhabitants of spaceship Earth. It was inevitable that this sort of mindset would encompass the issue of animal suffering at human hands. Indeed, many leaders in the crusade for a new ethic for animals are veterans of other social struggles—the civil rights, labor, and feminist movements. The treatment of animals is thus perceived as continuous with a wide variety of other socioethical concerns.

## The Rational Articulation of a Moral Base

Hegel once remarked that the job of philosophers was to articulate in an explicit and rational fashion currents of thought that were inchoately surfacing in society in general. Beginning in the 1970s, philosophers have done just that with regard to the social ethic for animals. Departing from the traditional twentieth-century tendency of philosophers to talk only to other philosophers, some have spoken to society at large and helped shape and draw out the emerging ethic for animals. Significantly, few philosophers have defended the status quo regarding animal use; one who did so, Michael A. Fox, who wrote a moral defense of animal use in research, rapidly repudiated his own argument.[17]

Many of these philosophers have addressed their remarks to the general public, garnering a good deal of attention. Peter Singer's seminal *Animal Liberation* has been steadily in print since 1975; my own *Animal Rights and Hu-*

*man Morality* has been in print since 1981; both works are in second editions. Such efforts, along with those of scientists, attorneys, and other professionals concerned about the issues, have done much to provide a rational framework for what would otherwise be unfocused and uninformed moral indignation and sentiment.

## The Nature of the Emerging Ethic: Beyond Cruelty

As Plato clearly explained, ethical change in society does not occur ex nihilo. One cannot simply enunciate a new ethic and expect it to take hold and flourish. That is why Plato said that moral philosophers cannot *teach* but can only *remind*. If a person or a society is to be persuaded to change morally, it will be because the change elaborates, expands on, or unpacks some moral principle that the person or society already holds. To be sure, persons or societies may not be clear about what they believe or about the implications of what they believe; clarification becomes the job for those who deal with ethics$_2$.

Another way to express the same point can be drawn from physical combat. When one is obliged to fight a stronger opponent, it is foolhardy to pit one's inferior force against his superior force in a sumo encounter, a direct clash. A wiser strategy is to employ judo, directing the opponent's own force against him. The same holds true in ethics. If I oppose my moral position against yours in a frontal attack, I will have little chance of moving you from your entrenched position. If, however, I show you that my ideas are really yours, that is, are implicit in beliefs you already hold, I have much more of a chance of changing your mind.

Likewise, forcing a change in social ethics for which there is no implicit basis is guaranteed to fail. The passage and failure of Prohibition provides a superb historical example of forcing change not tied to prior beliefs about right and wrong. Few people in society—certainly nowhere near a consensus—believed that the consumption of alcohol was wrong. Nor were they committed to other beliefs that logically entailed that drinking alcohol was wrong. Prohibition had absolutely no point of contact with extant morality and hence had no effect. A similar case is the communist government's attempt to ban religious life in Poland. The ban merely drove religion underground and probably strengthened people's religious commitments.

On the other hand, remarkable changes in social ethics have occurred where there is an implicit basis for them. One of the best illustrations is provided by Lyndon Johnson's passage of the Civil Rights Act. Johnson, an astute judge of character and a Southerner, believed that most people who explicitly discriminated against blacks nonetheless would acquiesce to the following assumptions inherent in our democratic theory:

> All humans should be treated equally.
> Blacks are humans.
> Separate is not equal.

Such people had just never extracted or noticed the implication of their own assumptions. By "writing this large" in law, Johnson realized one could get people to recollect and, albeit reluctantly, work toward the abolition of institutionalized discrimination.

Any new ethic for animals, therefore, in order to garner widespread social acquiescence, would have to draw on moral principles already there. And this is precisely what has taken place.

As we have seen, society has grown increasingly concerned about animal suffering even when the source of the suffering is not cruelty, most notably in the case of research and confinement agriculture, but also in such areas as trapping. Indeed, a 1985 case in New York State vividly pointed out the need for ethical evolution beyond cruelty.[18] A group of attorneys brought suit against the branch of New York State government charged with administering public lands on the grounds that the agency's permitting the use of steel-jawed traps on public lands entailed violation of the cruelty laws, since animals so trapped were deprived of food, water, and medical care for injury. Although sympathetic to the moral point, the judge dismissed the case, reiterating that the cruelty laws did not apply to "standard" practices such as trapping, which fulfill a legal human purpose—provision of furs and pest control. If the plaintiffs wished to ban steel-jawed traps, said the judge, they needed to go to the legislature, that is, change the social ethic, not to the judiciary, which is bound by the ethic encoded in the anticruelty laws.

Thus, society is faced with the need for new moral categories and laws that reflect those categories in order to deal with animal use in science and agriculture and to limit the animal suffering with which it is increasingly concerned. At the same time, society has gone through almost fifty years of extending its moral categories for *humans* to people who were morally ignored or invisible. As noted, new and viable ethics₁ does not emerge ex nihilo. So a plausible and obvious move is for society to continue in its tendency and *attempt to extend the moral machinery it has developed for dealing with people, appropriately modified, to animals.* And this is precisely what has occurred. Society has taken elements of the moral categories it uses for assessing the treatment of people and is in the process of modifying these concepts to make them appropriate for dealing with new issues in the treatment of animals, especially their use in science and confinement agriculture.

What aspect of our ethic for people is being so extended? One that is, in fact, quite applicable to animal use. All human communities face a fundamental problem of weighing the interests of the individual against those of the general welfare. Different societies have provided different answers to this problem. Totalitarian societies opt to devote little concern to the individual, favoring instead the state, or whatever their version of the general welfare may be. At the other extreme, anarchical groups such as communes give primacy to the individual and very little concern to the group—hence they tend to enjoy only transient existence. In our society, however, a balance is struck. Although most of our decisions are made to the benefit of the general welfare, fences are built around individuals to protect their fundamental interests from being sacrificed to the majority. Thus we protect individuals from being silenced even if the majority disapproves of what they say; we protect individuals from having their property seized without recompense even if such seizure benefits the general welfare; we protect individuals from torture even if they have planted a bomb in an elementary school and refuse to divulge its location. We protect those interests of the individual that we consider essential to being human, to *human nature,* from being submerged, even by the common good. Those moral/legal fences that so protect the individual human are called *rights* and are based on plausible assumptions regarding what is essential to being human.

It is this notion to which society in general is looking in order to generate the new moral notions necessary to talk about the treatment of animals in today's world, where cruelty is not the major problem but where such laudable, general welfare goals as efficiency, productivity, knowledge, medical progress, and product safety are responsible for the vast majority of animal suffering. People are seeking to "build fences" around animals to protect them and their interests and natures from being totally submerged for the sake of the general welfare, and are following the New York judge's advice to accomplish this goal by going to the legislature.

It is necessary to stress here certain things that this ethic, in its mainstream version, is *not* and does not attempt to be. As a mainstream movement, it does not try to give human rights to animals. Since animals do not have the same natures and interests flowing from these natures as humans do, human rights do not fit animals. Animals do not have basic natures that demand speech, religion, or property; thus according them these rights would be absurd. On the other hand, animals have natures of their own (what I have, following Aristotle, called their *telos*)[19] and interests that flow from these natures, and the thwarting of these interests matters to animals as much as the thwarting of speech matters to humans. The agenda is not, for mainstream society, making animals "equal" to people. It is rather preserving the common-sense insight that "fish gotta swim and birds gotta fly," and suffer if they don't.

Nor is this ethic, in the minds of mainstream society, an abolitionist one, dictating that animals cannot be used by humans. Rather, it is an attempt to constrain *how* they can be used, so as to limit their pain and suffering. In this regard, as a 1993 *Beef Today* article points out,[20] the thrust for protection of animal natures is not at all radical; it is very conservative, *asking for the same sort of husbandry that characterized the overwhelming majority of animal use during all of human history, save the last fifty or so years.* It is not opposed to animal use; it is opposed to animal use that goes against the animals' natures and tries to force square pegs into round holes, leading to friction and suffering. If animals are to be used for food and labor, they should, as they traditionally did, live lives that respect their natures. If animals are to be used to probe nature and cure disease for human benefit, they should not suffer in the process. Thus this new ethic is conservative, not radical, harking back to the animal use that necessitated and thus entailed respect for the animals' natures. It is based on the insight that what we do to animals *matters* to them, just as what we do to humans matters to them, and that consequently we should respect that mattering in our treatment and use of animals as we do in our treatment and use of humans. And since respect for animal nature is no longer automatic as it was in traditional agriculture, society is demanding that it be encoded in law.

Granted, there are activists who do not wish to see animals used in any way by humans, and in the eyes of many animal users, the activists *are* the "animal rights people." Yet to focus on them is to eclipse the main point of the animal rights thrust in society in general—it is an effort to constrain *how* we use animals, not an attempt to stop all animal use. Indeed, it is only in the context of animal use that constraints on use make any sense at all! Thus the new mainstream ethic is not an ethic of abolition; it is an effort to reaffirm that the interests of the animals count for themselves, not only in terms of how they benefit us. And like all rights ethics, it accepts that some benefits to be gained by unbridled exploitation will be lost and that there is a cost to protecting the animals' natures. In agriculture, for example, the cost may be higher food prices. But as the Federation of European Veterinarians asserted, that is a small price for a society to pay to ensure proper treatment of objects of moral concern.

Thus, the new animal rights ethic we have described in society in general should not be viewed as radically different from concerns about animal welfare, as agriculturalists often mistakenly do. It is, in fact, the *form* that welfare concerns are taking in the face of what has occurred in science and agriculture since World War II. The demand for rights fills the gap left by the loss of traditional husbandry agriculture and its built-in guarantee of protection of fundamental animal interests.

## Evidence for the Presence of the New Ethic

The presence of the ethic in mainstream society is not difficult to document. A 1989 *Parents* magazine survey indicated that 80 percent of its readership (mainstream, middle-class people) believed that animals had rights, while 84 percent believed we could use animals for food.[21] For almost a decade, roughly the early 1980s into the 1990s, Congress received more letters on animal welfare–related issues than on any others.[22] Scores of bills are introduced into local, state, and federal legislatures every year pertaining to animal welfare in all areas of human use of animals, most of which were traditionally unregulated, from animal research to zoos. Traditional hurtful uses of animals have been modified in a variety of areas. Zoos have been working to provide environments that meet the needs of animals' natures, as have aquaria. In one case, the Canadian Ministry of Fisheries and Oceans would not allow the Vancouver Aquarium to take a killer whale from Canadian waters for exhibition until the aquarium had demonstrated that it could house the animal in such a way as to allow it to express its nature. The European Community has made concern about farm animal welfare a major priority, as have numerous European countries. Most notable is Sweden, which in 1988 passed what the *New York Times* called an "animal rights law,"[23] disallowing confinement agriculture based on efficiency alone and mandating that the rearing of animals be suited to the animals' natures. The law moved through the Swedish Parliament virtually unopposed and was perceived by the Swedish public not as radical but as a return to traditional agricultural values of husbandry. The same conceptual-ethical point was made by the Brambell Commission in Great Britain when it was chartered in 1965 in response to widespread public concern about confinement agriculture.

In the United States, the most obvious effect of the new ethic has been in the area of animal use in scientific research. Despite vigorous opposition from the powerful and wealthy biomedical community, two pieces of federal legislation, reflective of the new ethic, were passed in 1985, placing significant constraints on animal use in a field that had historically enjoyed laissez-faire in this area. The story of this legislation, which is discussed shortly, is highly germane to the issue of farm animal welfare and should serve as an object lesson to the agricultural community.

It is clear that the next area of animal use for which society is likely to demand legislation is agriculture. In the early 1990s, Representative Charles Stenholm of Texas, a member of the House Agriculture Committee and a solid spokesman for agriculture, predicted that legislation aimed at ensuring farm animal welfare could be promulgated by the year 2000 if the industry fails to respond to these concerns. It thus behooves the agricultural community to heed the lessons of what has occurred in the biomedical area, for as George Santayana remarked, those who cannot remember the past are condemned to repeat it. Since the author was personally involved in drafting the legislation dealing with animal research, as well as in shepherding it through Congress and defending it against hostile criticism from both the research and the radical animal rights community, he is in a unique position to reflect upon its implications for the related issue of agricultural animal welfare.

As already mentioned, the scientific community had traditionally enjoyed unrestricted autonomy in the care and use of research animals. As in agriculture, the anticruelty laws specifically exempted research activities from their purview. Furthermore, as the research community argued, animal research had produced significant benefits for society: drugs, operative procedures, new therapeutic modalities. Thus, during the ascendance of the traditional ethic proscribing cruelty, society had little cause to question such research uses, as scientists were manifestly not guilty of cruelty, that is, deliberate, useless infliction of pain. Indeed, before the 1960s, scientists were culturally perceived as folk heroes.

Beginning in the 1960s, however, public disenchantment with science and technology began to grow, a trend that has greatly concerned the scientific community.[24] The war on cancer did not defeat cancer; technology was blamed for environmental despoliation and degradation (science and technology are not always distinguished in the public mind); revelations of abuse of human and animal subjects proliferated; scientists were caught misappropriating grant money and falsifying data. Social concern about animal treatment naturally gravitated toward research, which most people found alien and remote. Publicity about kidnapping of pets for research and about poor conditions under which dog dealers kept animals led to the 1966 Animal Welfare Act, passed largely to assuage fears of pet owners about their animals being kidnapped and sold to research laboratories. Rats, mice, birds, and farm animals were exempted from any protection, though standards for husbandry and caging were promulgated for other animals.

The research community remained mostly unaffected by the act in its day-to-day practices and continued to give issues of animal care low priority, still assuming that the public would care only about the results of research, not about the animals. By the late 1970s, however, the new ethic for animals had grown sufficiently that large portions of the public wanted assurance that research animals were indeed not suffering uncontrolled pain and were receiving proper care. The research community still misunderstood the moral basis of the social concern and continued to advocate for unrestricted animal use in utilitarian terms, arguing that any constraints on animal use would jeopardize the curing of disease (despite the fact that evidence garnered by Congress demonstrated that cavalier treatment of animals compromised research results).[25]

In the mid-1970s, a group of Colorado citizens, mostly scientists and veterinarians representing more than fifty years of animal research experience, and including an attorney and a philosopher (myself), began to think through legislation that would protect animals while not stifling science; indeed, it was our belief that legislated standards for proper treatment would *ensure* good science by eliminating variables introduced into experiments by uncontrolled stress and pain. For example, in the case of animals used in cancer research, if the animals were not treated well, one could not tell whether their tumors were the result of the substances being tested or the result of stressful conditions.[26]

Our approach was to mandate "enforced self-regulation" by stipulating some general principles and requiring local institutional committees to oversee and enforce them. The principles were simple:

1. Animals should not suffer pain or distress unless the pain or distress was the object of the experiment, or unless the control of pain and distress would compromise the results. (These exceptions apply to only about 10 percent of animal research protocols.)

2. Animals should not be used repeatedly for invasive experiments.

3. Paralytics (drugs which cause paralysis but leave the animals fully conscious) should not be used without general anesthesia.

4. Husbandry and housing should fit the animals' natures.

5. Local committees of scientists and nonscientists should oversee the foregoing principles through review of scientific protocols inspection of facilities.

Our proposals were not embraced by the research community, despite the fact that growing social concern for research animals was manifest and evidence of poor animal treatment continued to mount. We were denounced as radicals; I was called an "apologist for lab trashers" and an "exonerator of the Nazis" in the *New England Journal of Medicine*.[27] At the same time, I was called a "sell-out" for "accepting the reality of science" by animal rights extremists.

Nonetheless, by 1985, our proposal had been translated into two pieces of federal legislation, one an amendment to the Animal Welfare Act, the other a mandate to the National Institutes of Health (NIH). By that time, a significant portion of the research community had accepted our approach, in large part because public support for another law—the Research Modernization Act, which would have cut the federal research budget by up to 60 percent and plowed that amount into the study of alternatives to the use of research animals—was steadily increasing. Our group went from being characterized as antiscience and antiresearch to being seen as, in the words of one high NIH official, "the salvation of biomedicine."

It is now clear to the research community that we were correct on four counts:

1. The public wanted assurance of proper care and treatment and pain control for animals used in research, not abolition of animal research. The public also did not believe that such a demand would cripple science.

2. The law provided such assurance.

3. The law helped promote good research, not hinder it.

4. The law helped accelerate proper animal care (for example, pain control) that was unlikely to develop otherwise.

Only our fourth principle, about care and housing fitting the animals' natures, was not fully adopted into law. Instead, the law mandated "exercise for dogs" and environments for primates that "enhance their psychological well-being." Other species are still generally housed in accordance with researcher convenience, though more thought is being directed at creating "animal-friendly" environments; an entire issue of *Lab Animal,* a trade journal, was recently devoted to enriched environments for nonmandated species.

Thus, the new ethic shaped these revolutionary laws governing biomedicine in a number of ways. First, the use of animals in research does not in and of itself ensure, as did traditional agriculture, that animals are relatively happy and are not suffering pain and distress. Second, at the same time, the pain and suffering experienced by research animals is not the result of cruelty. Third, society has embodied its demand for control of pain and suffering in the consensus ethic, at no little expense. (It is estimated that ensuring compliance with the 1985 amendment to the Animal Welfare Act alone has cost $500 million between 1985 and 1995.) Concern for the animals supersedes human utilitarian (economic) considerations. The right not to suffer in the course of being used for human benefit is thus encoded into law, as are the right to exercise for dogs and the right to a stimulating environment for primates. Fourth, virtually all animals used in biomedical research, with the exception of rodents and birds used in private industrial research, are covered by law. And in 1992, a federal judge declared that exemption of rodents from protection of the Animal Welfare Act by USDA regulations implementing the act violates the intent of the act.[28] Finally, the law is not abolitionist: it does not intend in any way to stop animal use in science but simply guarantees that animal suffering is controlled as far as possible.

## The Relevance of the New Social Ethic to Agriculture

It is important that those involved in animal agriculture fully understand the lesson implicit in the foregoing discussion of animal research and the new social ethic. The view that it is permissible to use animals for research, so long as there exist certain guarantees that the animals' fundamental interests are protected, can be extrapolated to agriculture. While the public accepts and demands animal products, it wants assurance that the animals are not miserable and indeed are happy. A 1991 survey reported by the National Cattlemen's Association indicates that although the majority of the public believes that stockmen take good care of their animals, an even greater percentage wish to see such treatment legislated.[29] The lesson is obvious.

Furthermore, both the mass media and the animal advocate organizations are actively involved in calling public attention to farm animal welfare issues and are gathering strength by linking animal welfare to environmental and food-safety issues. The following animal advocate organizations have specifically targeted the farm animal issue:

Animal Welfare Institute
Humane Society of the United States
Animal Rights International
Animal Legal Defense Fund
Animal Rights Network-*Agenda* Magazine
People for the Ethical Treatment of Animals
Action for Life
Association of Veterinarians for Animal Rights
Farm Animal Reform Movement
Farm Animal Concerns Trust
Humane Farming Association
Physicians Committee for Reform of Medicine
Farm Sanctuary[30]

U.S. society is extremely naive about the nature of agricultural production. Contrary to the beliefs of some elements of the agricultural community, however, it will not help to "educate" the public. In fact, if the public knew more about the way in which agricultural animal production infringes on animal welfare, the outcry would be louder. For example, in Saskatoon, Saskatchewan, a mid-sized city located in an agricultural area and thus not putatively agriculturally naive, 75 percent of the public believed that castration of beef cattle was done under anesthesia.[31] Another example is Frank Perdue's "happy chickens." Plainly, if the public knew, for instance, that some swine raised in total confinement literally never see the light of day, it would be more, not less, hostile to current agriculture. What, then, is to be done?

The agricultural and agricultural research communities have a window of opportunity, comparable to the one that was available to the research community in the late 1970s, to show the public that they recognize the welfare problems in current agriculture and are addressing them in a meaningful way. This may mean that the agricultural community should develop its own legislation before uninformed legislation is thrust on it. (Legislation may be necessary both to reassure the public and to level the playing field for all producers.) It certainly means that the agricultural community should proactively take up the problem areas in confinement agriculture as well as in such traditional agriculture as range beef production so as to harmonize all agricultural production with the new ethic.

Such attention must focus on all the sources of animal suffering we discussed earlier: production diseases, lack of individual attention, and, most important, the failure of intensive systems to allow animals to actualize their telos, that is, their biological/psychological natures. In addition, sources of suffering independent of intensive agriculture should be addressed: shipping, rough handling, downer animals, and invasive practices such as castration, branding, and dehorning that are relevant to extensively managed animals.

Clearly, the most difficult challenge to agriculture is accommodating the animals' natures in intensive systems. It is socially and economically impossible to return completely to fully extensive but husbandry-oriented management systems for farm animals, except for relatively small portions of the producer community that wish to exploit niche markets. (The size of this niche should itself be studied.) On the other hand, as we see in Part 2, certain animals can be raised under semi-extensive conditions profitably—swine, for example. For the rest of agriculture, the challenge is to make intensive systems "animal-friendly," that is, to create systems that satisfy animals' psychological/biological natures, and the interests flowing therefrom, yet are economically viable.

In this endeavor the U.S. agricultural community is not starting from zero. Canada, the Netherlands, Switzerland, Britain, and especially Sweden have undertaken research into such alternatives for some time. These countries have been more sensitized to the welfare issues than the United States, since they experienced their change in public sentiment earlier. U.S. agriculture should learn from their mistakes and successes.

Animal welfare–friendly agriculture is a viable area of research. All parties to the debate see research as a necessary way of moving forward and finding solutions. In particular, research should be directed at all the sources of animal suffering in agriculture, whether or not they are associated with intensive agriculture. But it is clearly research into meeting the behavioral and psychological needs of animals which is most demanded by the new ethic and yet is most difficult for agriculturalists and agricultural scientists to carry out.

At the Maryland Conference on Farm Animal Welfare in 1991, Stanley Curtis pointed out that the development of confinement agriculture after World War II had been driven by a circumscribed set of values—the production of cheap and plentiful food. At that time, he argued, no one was talking about the ethological, behavioral, or psychological needs of farm animals, so these considerations did not enter into the reckoning of those who contrived intensive systems. Now that the public demands that such needs be addressed, however, it must allow the agricultural community time to build them into extant or modified confinement systems. Such change cannot occur overnight.[32]

There is a good deal of truth in these remarks. But the public, if aroused, will demand immediate action, which may cause harm to producers without benefiting animals. In this regard, it is worth recalling what occurred in the area of biomedicine. While the biomedical community continued to resist even the enforced self-regulation we had drafted, the public became increasingly convinced of the need for regulation of biomedical research, and the passage of legislation became more likely. In comparison to the Research Modernization Act, our legislation became more attractive to the research community. Thus, by the time I was called on to testify before the House Subcommittee on Health and Environment on behalf of the Walgren version of our bill in 1982, I carried the endorsement of the American Physiological Society, the traditional *opponent* of any intrusion into the research process.

The agriculture community, in my view, can still take the initiative in addressing the issue of farm animal welfare. No significant proposals for legislation or even demand for the regulation of confinement agriculture have yet emerged from animal welfare interests. They cannot conceive what form such legislation could take. Such a demand could be quickly galvanized, however, in response to high-visibility news stories regarding confinement agriculture. The 1990 videotapes of downer cattle at the Minneapolis–South St. Paul stockyards provide a small example of the way in which media exposure of animal abuse can rapidly generate demand for legislation—indeed, legislation forbidding marketing of downer cattle is still very much alive as of this writing.[33]

The agricultural and the agricultural research communities must therefore proactively and immediately undertake research that directly addresses improving the welfare of farm animals and then publicize such activities and the results. The research should be funded by both the government and the industry. In this way, the industry can assure the public that it is aware of the problems and is working to solve them. A failure to provide such assurance could lead to a rapid erosion of public confidence in the industry, creating a vacuum that could be filled by hasty and ill-considered legislation. The presence of meaningful, ongoing research devoted to improving the welfare of farm animals can even blunt the political effect of sensational news coverage of abuses associated with production agriculture. The public is not stupid. If it believes that government and industry are genuinely and demonstrably addressing and researching the issues of farm animal welfare in ways it can understand, it can probably be persuaded to allow the industry the time necessary to effect change. If, on the other hand, the industry cannot cite evidence of meaningful research efforts, the public could well demand precipitous action. If public concern accelerates to that point, the agriculture community can tie such legislation to the research progress it has achieved in making confinement agriculture more animal-friendly and project the amount of time needed to change the industry without disastrous results.

Thus, government and industry must not only undertake research, *but undertake research that meshes with public concerns and with the ethic that has emerged.* Society will no longer be satisfied with research far removed from viable solutions; endlessly measuring cortisol, for example, will not protect the industry. For research to be successful in reassuring the public, it should assume that animals can suffer in a variety of ways; be primarily directed at alleviating that suffering, not attempting to prove that it does not exist; and be compatible with the social ethic we have described, not profess to be independent of social values. The luxury of pure research not clearly understood to be tied to animal welfare will not be enough to satisfy socioethical concerns.

The area of research animal use should again serve as a model. Before the advent of federal legislation, the research community had an ideological stance against accepting the reality of felt pain and suffering in animals as part of the legitimate purview of scientific study. Anthropomorphic extrapolations from human to animal were summarily rejected. Yet the federal laws simply asserted that animals felt pain and that anthropomorphic extrapolations *were* legitimate. Public attitudes toward the reality and moral relevance of animal pain and suffering thus provided the ground rules according to which both research and legislation regulating research were played out. The same is undoubtedly true of farm animal welfare and research relevant to improving and ensuring such welfare. In other words, research designed to accommodate public moral concern about farm animal welfare and alleviation of pain and suffering must be consonant with these attitudes, not at loggerheads with them.

Finally, before research of the sort we have just discussed can be successfully undertaken, the scientists who will carry it out must be educated to its basic purpose—alleviating public concern about farm animal welfare. Without such education, scientists will be too academic and insufficiently pragmatic in their approach to the research program. Steps must be taken to ensure that the research undertaken will directly address the socioethical issues that prompted it in the first place.

# 2 Welfare Research and Scientific Ideology

## Scientific and Producer Attitudes toward Animal Welfare

Certain features of the attitude of both the agricultural producer community and the agricultural science community must be revised or eliminated before the sort of research we have sketched can be done—and publicized—in such a way as to satisfy the general public that agriculture is making a genuine effort to meet social ethical concerns about animals. These features tend to distance the mindset of those chartering and doing the research from that of the general public and thus blunt the effectiveness of any research efforts. Such counterproductive elements of thought are variously held by producers and scientists, and both groups must carefully consider why they are best abandoned. The problematic beliefs are as follows:

1. The view that animal welfare and animal rights represent a clear-cut dichotomy, separated by an unbridgeable gulf. Animal welfare is perceived as an acceptable concern of producers; animal rights is denied any legitimacy. This opinion is held strongly by producers, agricultural scientists, and veterinarians and is essentially never questioned.

2. The conviction that one can talk of animal welfare in a value-free, objective, factual context. Again, this view is held by all elements of agriculture but is elicited most easily from scientists, who are steeped in the belief that science is value-free.

3. The general principle that science and ethics are radically separated, with science having no connection to ethics.

4. The notion that research into animal welfare cannot address, in any scientific way, issues pertaining to animal consciousness or animal feeling, including felt pain and suffering.[1]

These four beliefs are inextricably intertwined and can usually be separated only conceptually. Nonetheless, they collectively create a barrier to agricultural research into animal welfare, even if such research is well funded (which it currently is not) and comprehensive. We therefore discuss each one in detail.

## The Alleged Cleavage between Animal Welfare and Animal Rights

The agricultural community's general attitude toward the difference between animal welfare and animal rights was pithily summed up by one of my colleagues in animal science when he asserted, "Too often, the ag community takes this position: Animal welfare is what we already do; animal rights is what *they* want us to do!" In other words, "Animal welfare, *sí;* animal rights, no!" Animal welfare is perceived as the purview of "responsible" people; animal rights is seen as the domain of the radical fringe.

As our discussion thus far has indicated, this view is simply incorrect factually. Certainly there are fringe groups, extremists, who argue that animals are morally no different from people and that all animal use is immoral. (Indeed, their counterparts exist on the other side, people who maintain that there should be no constraints whatever on human treatment of animals. I have heard this put, for example, as "God said we could do whatever we wish with animals.")

But we have also seen that the majority of people believe that animals have rights *and* that humans may use animals. Of the approximately seven to ten thousand western ranchers with whom I have discussed this issue in detail, between 80 and 95 percent also affirm that animals have rights in the sense we discussed earlier. It is likely that most animal agriculturalists in general would share this view; that, at least, has been my experience with swine producers, dairy producers, and cattle feeders and other agriculturalists across the English-speaking world.

Thus, if it is the case that the notion of animal rights is a pivotal part of the emerging mainstream social ethic for the treatment of animals, there is little value in maintaining the dualism of animal welfare versus animal rights. It is rather that the traditional notion of animal welfare is being socially augmented and explicated by the notion that animals have certain rights.

## The View that Welfare Is Value-Free

The sharp cleavage between animal welfare and animal rights has, in turn, been reinforced by the common belief that the concept of "welfare" is (or can be) a purely factual notion, devoid of any moral or otherwise valuational content. One can thus find a widespread belief in agriculture, and among agricultural scientists especially, that one can study animal welfare without any appeal to or reliance on ethical notions. Indeed, if one searches the major scientific/industry literature on farm animal welfare, one finds a radical distancing of the "scientific" concept of welfare from any ethical dimensions.

Such an approach is, for example, trumpeted in the passage chartering the American Veterinary Medical Association Animal Welfare Committee, where it was proclaimed that "AVMA positions should be concerned primarily with the scientific aspects of the medical well-being of animals, rather than the philosophical or moral aspects."[2] It is echoed in the preface to a report of the Council for Agricultural Science and Technology (CAST), appropriately entitled *Scientific Aspects of the Welfare of Food Animals,* which "focuses primarily on the welfare of food animals. ... The Animal Rights issue has to do with human ethics and not with science; consequently it is not addressed at length."[3] More specific suggestions, such as that of Cambridge ethologist Donald Broom, who defines welfare as adaptation to or coping with the environment, also eschew any commitment to moral values.[4] Even the most sophisticated views of animal welfare, such as those offered by Marian Dawkins or Ian Duncan,[5] which accept the reality of animal subjective experience, presuppose the conceptual separability of animal welfare science and ethical judgments, with scientists supplying value-free data and society making ethical judgments.

A moment's reflection will, of course, reveal that the concept of welfare is at root valuational. Most simply, the choice of what facts to count as relevant to an animal's welfare is determined by one's values, not merely by the facts. When producers talk of animal welfare, they use one set of facts to determine its presence or absence; when the general public, or animal advocates, talk of animal welfare, they look to another set of facts as relevant.

Specifically, by *welfare,* producers mean the presence of conditions relevant to the purposes for which the animal is raised. The animal receives food, water, shelter, protection from predators, and so on, all of which allow it to thrive in terms of the producer's purpose for the animal—being sold for food or producing products sold for food. Even treatment or prevention of disease enters into this view only insofar as it is relevant to the animal's productivity, or, even more tellingly, insofar as it is relevant to the productivity of the whole operation. Thus, as we saw, those production diseases that are reckoned inevitable consequences of efficient production systems, such as liver abscesses in cattle, may be simply accepted as part of the price of the system. In other words, in a contemporary agricultural context, the role and value of animals are defined in terms of their economic efficiency and productivity (and the prices for their products). In this valuational context, animal welfare (and its study) is restricted to what has an effect on production and price. This approach is graphically illustrated in a letter I recently saw from a government agricultural official supporting the establishment of a chair in animal welfare at a university. The official wrote that he favored "the development of definitive criteria in assessing the amount of stress that animals are undergoing and the compatibility of the stress with the animal's productive life."

In contrast, nonproducers—that is, the general public—may worry about animal boredom, social deprivation, or psychological well-being as relevant to animal welfare, even though these factors may be irrelevant to (i.e., have no impact on) productivity or may decrease efficiency by raising costs of production.

Thus what the producer counts as data or facts relevant to whether the animals are in states of positive or negative welfare differs from what the animal advocate or person in the street so counts (though there is some significant overlap between the two). This dispute cannot be decided simply by appeal to facts; rather, *what we count as facts relevant to the issue is decided by our concept of welfare, which, in turn, depends in large part on what we consider worth worrying about (valuing) regarding how the animal lives its life.*

Once we decide what we value as relevant to, or constitutive of, welfare, we can appeal to facts supporting its presence or absence in a given instance. But whether we decide to use a concept of welfare or well-being that looks at production criteria alone or one that also counts what the animal experiences is determined by our ethical stance relative to the animal.

A major reason that this point has been ignored is the general view, widespread among scientists, that science is value-free. But another reason can be found in our earlier discussion. In traditional agriculture, there was a much closer fit between the two diverse concepts of welfare just enumerated. Under extensive conditions, if one met the animal's needs relevant to production, one was much more likely to meet the needs associated with the animal's psychological nature as well; the needs for companionship, a stimulating environment, and the like were satisfied by grazing a herd on the range, for example. But in technological agriculture, one can meet one set of needs without necessarily meeting the others, giving rise to the splitting of the notion of welfare into multiple concepts that are counted or not, depending on one's values.

Another argument can be marshaled to show that there is a variety of valuational notions implicit in the concept of welfare. One of the simplest yet most compelling ways of buttressing this claim is to point to the relevance of health and disease to the concept of animal welfare. However many divergent definitions of animal welfare one may encounter in the literature, surely all would consider health an essential part of welfare, and disease an indication against the presence of welfare. But when one begins to think carefully about health and disease, one realizes that even these basic concepts are inextricably bound up with value judgments, including moral ones. Health is not merely statistical normality and disease statistical abnormality, for what is statistically normal in a population may well be what we consider disease, and what we call healthy may be statistically rare. Rather, health and disease are based in a complex set of values, including ethical ones.[6] The World Health Organization's definition of health as a "complete state of physical, mental, and social well-being" strikingly illustrates this point, as do recent medical pronouncements that child abuse, spousal abuse, alcoholism, and obesity are sicknesses to be treated, not bad behavior to be punished.

As I have shown elsewhere,[7] what counts as medically real in animals (i.e., worthy of being treated) is not only what science finds but what society considers significant. When the role and value of animals in society are overwhelmingly economic, symptoms, syndromes, discomfort, or abnormality that have no apparent relevance to animal productivity, to survival as presuppositional to productivity, to marketability, or to other human uses for the animal do not become medically real—hence, the ignoring of animal pain by science and veterinary medicine during most of the twentieth century.[8] The only time animal pain was implicitly recognized in science was when it served human ends, as when pain was induced in animals to test analgesics in humans. No one ever thought to worry about the animal pain per se and its control, and it was common to deny its reality. Anesthesia was called "chemical restraint." Food animal veterinarians typically did not (and still do not) worry about the pain of cattle castration, dehorning, branding, or other procedures; such a concern was not perceived as economically viable. Similarly, laboratory animal veterinarians did not worry about postsurgical pain in animals until society laws declared in the 1985 federal laws that control of such pain was part of their job. (As a result, more papers were produced on analgesia in animals in the ensuing six years than in the previous one hundred.)

Indeed, what I have elsewhere called the "physicalization of pain and stress,"[9] that is, the looking at and defining of pain and stress solely in terms of physiological processes rather than in terms of what the animal feels (even though the work of John Mason[10] and others had shown that what the animal experiences is highly relevant to the physical stress response), still pervasive in science, can only happen when society and science do not morally concern themselves about animal experience. Ordinary common sense has never denied that animals have a full range of subjective experiences; people just did not morally care about it until very recently, save for unnecessary pain and suffering inflicted by intentional cruelty.

In summary, if the concepts of health and disease are essential to the concept of animal welfare, and the concepts of health and disease are laden with ethical and other values, necessarily the notion of animal welfare is also so laden.

## The View that Science Is Value-Free

A common belief among scientists is that all of science is "value-free"; that science is, and ought to be, disengaged from any valuational presuppositions and commitments, and, even more so, removed from any moral values.[11] This position is, in turn, part of the general view of the nature of science that scientists have held throughout most of the twentieth century. Scientists acquire an account of the nature of science while they are beginning students, along with the facts of their discipline, and that account is constantly reinforced during their training years and in their professional lives. In and of itself, this is unexceptionable, since as Aristotle long ago pointed out, all practitioners of any pursuit begin with a certain set of assumptions about their discipline that is simply taken for granted as presuppositional. After all, one cannot prove everything, or else one is led to an infinite regression, so it is appropriate to begin, as we do in geometry, with certain assumptions. It is only when these assumptions are hardened into orthodoxy, impervious to criticism and held as dogma, that they become pernicious. Unfortunately, many of the assumptions made about science have been uncritically taken as absolute, so much so that it is fair to call them "scientific ideology" or the "common sense of science," as I have done elsewhere.[12]

The roots of scientific common sense were grounded in the desire to draw a clear distinction between genuine science and "softer" fields such as theology and philosophy, which in the nineteenth century had become mixed with science, for example, among biologists who appealed to "life force" to explain biological phenomena. Indeed, in Germany at least, the science of physics varied considerably from university to university, depending on the philosophical school that was dominant at a given institution. Thus there arose a commendable effort to excise such extraneous components from science. This effort took the form of attempting to excise from science any notions which could not be "cashed out experientially," and was articulated as the principle of verification by the influential school of philosopher-scientists called the logical positivists. According to this principle, no concepts could be admitted into science unless they could be tied directly to empirical observations. By the same token, no judgments were to be considered scientifically legitimate unless one could specify how they could be verified or falsified empirically. It was, indeed, adherence to something like this principle that led Einstein to reject Newtonian absolute space and absolute time and to develop the notion of special relativity.

Laudable though this program may have been, it ushered in some untoward consequences. As is so often the case with excisive programs, wheat was discarded along with chaff. Thus the dogma developed among scientists that science was "value-free" in general and "ethics-free" in particular. Since value judgments of any sort cannot be verified and falsified, the argument went, they had no relevance to science. All values were at best expressions of subjective feeling with no cognitive content. Ideologically shielded by the value-free dogma, science was able to proceed without reflection on ethical matters directly relevant to its activity.

Adherence to this belief can be found at all levels of scientific activity. Introductions to basic textbooks trumpet the allegedly value-free nature of science. W. T. Keeton and J. L. Gould, for example, in their widely used freshman biology text, remark that "science cannot make value judgments ... and cannot make moral judgments."[13] In the same vein, Sylvia Mader, in her basic biology text, asserts that "science does not make ethical or moral decisions."[14] This ideology persists at the highest level of scientific activity. For example, James Wyngaarden, former director of the National Institutes of Health, declared in 1989 that all the controversy about genetic engineering was misdirected, for "science should not be hampered by ethical judgments."[15]

The pernicious consequences of this doctrine are obvious, not least because it has led scientists to ignore socioethical concerns until they have reached critical mass in society in general. For example, as Jay Katz of Yale has documented, the medical research community failed to see the moral issues implicit in the use of human subjects for research until forced to address them by threat of legislation.[16] Similarly, this community had never addressed the multiplicity of moral issues associated with the use of animals in research and was thus blind-sided by the intensity and pervasiveness of society's demand for legislation ensuring moral concern for research animals.

This ideological barrier must be overcome if farm animal welfare research is to be truly relevant to the social concerns that are demanding such research. Such research is not "ethics-free"—it is quite frankly being directed by a morally based agenda, namely, to accommodate the emerging ethic we have described, while preserving the benefits of modern agriculture, and to accomplish this task in an economically viable way. Furthermore, such research must generate solutions expeditiously, at least with sufficient alacrity that the public does not, out of frustration, seek its own, unfounded answers to what it increasingly perceives as a pressing moral problem.

Equally important, the results of research into animal welfare must accord with the social concerns responsible for that research in the first place. And if researchers do not understand and assimilate the ethic, they will simply be unable to harness their research to it. For example, research that presupposes that we must be agnostic about whether animals are suffering in confinement, however well it may be done, will simply not do the job needed. Similarly, research that is predicated on the assumption that productivity alone should determine our choice of systems will not resolve social concern. Or again, research that purports to prove that veal calves, for example, are better off in crates will again not serve the public demand, nor will it benefit agriculture, for it will simply erode confidence in welfare research.

Little research into animal well-being has been funded in the twentieth century, either by government or by industry. To be sure, there was certainly a great deal of research that could be described as relevant to animal welfare—studies of disease control, nutrition, bruising, stress, and the like—but it was motivated by and oriented toward improving those features of animal life relevant to the values that informed mid–twentieth century agriculture, namely, efficiency and productivity, that is, producing cheap and plentiful food. Until relatively recently, social ethics permitted this approach, largely because the public was unaware that traditional husbandry had been supplanted, as we discussed above. Now that society is concerned about animal suffering in confinement, the demand for research informed by other values has accelerated.

Specifically, society is demanding that agriculture be modified to reduce suffering and to accommodate the physical *and* psychological needs of animals, as determined by their biological natures. The aim of research into animal welfare that will hitherto be undertaken, therefore, must be primarily to improve the well-being of animals, presumably within the constraints of economic reality. This, in turn, means that research should be directed toward making production systems "animal-friendly," so as to alleviate suffering and increase animal happiness. This nonnegotiable feature of social demand must provide the stage on which research is played out. In short, research into animal well-being must become a moral science, in the judicious eighteenth-century sense of the term, conducted according to and oriented toward the ethic for animals that we have delineated as pervasive in society. For welfare research to attempt to contravene that ethic in any way is to bite the hand that feeds it, to lose credibility for research as a viable pathway to resolving the issues, and very likely to radicalize further the social position on industrialized agriculture.

## Scientific Agnosticism Regarding Animal Awareness

There is another aspect of scientific ideology that could potentially jeopardize the role of welfare research as a way of accommodating the new social concerns about animal agriculture and the new social ethic that has both shaped and been refined by that concern. This aspect is scientific ideology's traditional agnosticism about the ability of science to study, or even admit scientifically the existence of, animal consciousness, awareness, mind, pain, and suffering (as subjective experiences rather than as purely physical states).

Just as scientific ideology denied the legitimacy of talking about value judgments, including ethical ones, in science, it also historically denied science's ability to discuss mental states or states of consciousness in humans or animals.[17] This tendency grew out of the same positivistic leanings that led scientific ideology to the claim that science is value-free. In the domain of awareness, the ideology asserted that one could not verify claims about mental states in humans *or* animals, that "mind" was not subject to observation or experimentation, and that mental talk should thus be banished from scientific discourse.

Thus, even though Darwin had reasonably argued that if morphological and physiological traits were phylogenetically continuous, so too were mental ones; had further held that one could study feelings, perceptions, and thought in animals; and had demonstrated how this could be done, by 1920 virtually all American scientists had banished mind from scientific legitimacy, despite their nearly universal commitment to evolutionary theory.[18] Both human and animal psychology shifted from the study of consciousness to the study of behavior, and the ideological rejection of mind was stridently trumpeted by the American movement known as behaviorism. J. B. Watson, father of behaviorism, came perilously close to affirming that "we don't have thoughts; we only think we do," and Gordon Alport, president of the American Psychological Association, lamented the total disregard for consciousness in the psychological community in his 1939 presidential address:

> So it comes about that after the initial take-off we, as psychological investigators, are permanently barred from the benefit and counsel of our ordinary perceptions, feelings, judgments, and intuitions. We are allowed to appeal to them neither for our method nor for our validations. So far as "method" is concerned, we are told that, because the subject is able to make his discriminations only after the alleged experience has departed, any inference of a subjectively unified experience on his part is both anachronistic and unnecessary. If the subject protests that it is evident to him that he had a rich and vivid experience that was not fully represented in his overt discriminations, he is firmly assured that what is vividly self-evident to him is no longer of interest to the scientific psychologist. It has been decided, to quote Boring, that "in any useful meaning of the term existence, private experience does not exist."[19]

If human consciousness was banished, one can easily see that animal consciousness would certainly suffer a similar fate.

The scientific legitimacy of talk about animal consciousness was denied also by opponents of behaviorism. So strong was the positivist flame that it consumed discussion of consciousness in animals in Europe as well, where Konrad Lorenz and Nikolaas Tinbergen were opposing behaviorism with the fledgling science of ethology, on the grounds that behaviorism ignored genetic and evolutionary determinants of behavior. Nonetheless, ethologists denied the legitimacy of talking about consciousness in animals, the one point in which they stressed their agreement with behaviorists. Lorenz spoke of appetite behavior in animals, not of appetite, to stress the need for eschewing mentalism; behavioral psychologists spoke of aversive behavior and negative reinforcers, not of felt pain; biologists were carried along by the same current.

The two components of scientific ideology, the denial of values in science and the methodological elimination of talk about consciousness, naturally reinforced each other and were in turn buttressed by other factors. In particular, the philosophical denial of scientific reality to thought and feeling in animals helped allay reservations scientists might have had about hurting animals in the pursuit of scientific goals. Interestingly, the same thing had occurred in the seventeenth century when Descartes declared that animals were machines with no souls, minds, or feelings, thereby reconciling in one master stroke the demand that animals not have souls with his belief that biology is a part of physics and with the requirements of a growing science of physiology impelled in its quest for knowledge to do what common sense called painful procedures to animals without anesthetics. No need to control the pain, said Cartesian physiologists, because it is not really experienced pain, merely mechanical response. So too in the twentieth century the study of animal pain became the study of mechanical responses, not of felt hurt. Similarly, "stress" became a catchall for what ordinary common sense would call suffering and misery in a variety of forms and was described purely mechanistically in terms of activation of the hypophysis (pituitary) adrenal axis and its effects, with any notion of experienced suffering suppressed as scientifically illegitimate.

Furthermore, while ordinary common sense never denied the reality and knowability of animal pain and thus was shocked by the common sense of science (when it knew about it), it was not morally shocked. For although ordinary common sense never denied pain and suffering in animals, it did not worry a great deal about them either. Too much of ordinary practice and economic life depended on inflicting "necessary" pain and suffering on animals to devote much moral attention to it. Equally important, as we saw, the major social use of animals, traditional agriculture, was correctly perceived by society as requiring good treatment for farmers to be successful. This cavalier disregard for the moral relevance of animal suffering was, as we saw, mirrored in the legal system, which accorded animals the status of property; proscribed only overt and intentional cruelty, which might endanger human beings; and turned a blind eye to "necessary," expedient, and usual suffering.

By the same token, although turn-of-the-century veterinary medicine was certainly Darwinian in not denying the existence of pain in animals, its sense of moral responsibility for controlling pain was reflective of that of society in general, as the following quotation from a 1906 surgery text illustrates:

> In veterinary surgery, anesthesia has no history. It is used in a kind of desultory fashion that reflects no great credit to the present generation of veterinarians. ... Many veterinarians of rather wide experience have never in a

whole lifetime administered a general anesthetic in performing their operations. It reflects greatly to the credit of the canine specialist, however, that he alone has adopted anesthesia to any considerable extent. ... Anesthesia in veterinary surgery today is a means of restraint and not an expedient to relieve pain. So long as an operation can be performed by forcible restraint ... the thought of anesthesia does not enter into the proposition.[20]

Thus, for most of the century, ignoring animal pain, suffering, and the ethical dimensions of animal research were supported not only by a general social disregard for these issues and by a hard-fought tradition of academic freedom, but also by a ubiquitous and powerful ideology that said that science had no connection with values and that talk of animal mentation was operationally, empirically, scientifically meaningless. Only in such an environment could routine use of paralytics without anesthesia for some surgery (e.g., horse castration) flourish uncriticized, as it indeed did in research and veterinary practice.

Before 1985, there were virtually no scientific papers on animal analgesia or animal pain, though paradoxically, animals were used as models of human pain and to test analgesics. (It never occurred to scientific ideology that such use was tantamount to admitting that animals experienced felt pain or else they would not be valid research models!) When pain was addressed in animals, it was discussed in physicalistic, neurophysiological terms, not as a noxious subjective experience. "Stress" was explicated purely physiologically, generally in terms of activation of the pituitary adrenal axis for long-term stress and release of catecholamines for short-term stress. Alternatively, stress was described as anomalous and abnormal behavior, that is, stereotypies such as wind-sucking, cribbing (purposeless biting coupled with swallowing of air), pacing, bar-biting, weaving, and vacuum chewing (compulsive chewing even when nothing is ingested).

Animal science literature was especially guilty of treating stress purely physicalistically, as it became known that stress impaired productivity by leading to decreased immune function, greater disease susceptibility, weight loss, undesirable behaviors, lower reproductive success, and impaired products (e.g., "dark cutters" in beef and "pale, exudative, soft" meat in pork). The papers presented in 1982 at the first conference on animal pain, later published as *Animal Pain* by the American Physiological Society,[21] were, with a few notable exceptions, aimed at exploring the "plumbing of pain," that is, mechanisms of pain response. They tended to avoid moral issues involved in pain infliction and control and the fundamental morally relevant experiential dimension of pain: the fact that the animal *hurts*.

It was social moral concern for animals used in research that forced the biomedical research community both to deal with ethical issues and to reappropriate ordinary common sense with regard to animal consciousness and feeling. When the public demanded that animals used in research not experience suffering, pain, or distress, the research community quickly learned that it could not respond by denying their reality. As David Hume pointed out in the eighteenth century, and as the AVMA Panel on Pain and Distress of 1987 echoed, "no truth appears ... more evident than that beasts are endowed with thought and reason as well as men. The arguments are in this case so obvious, that they never escape the most stupid and ignorant."[22] Baldly put, in the face of social policy that legally compels ethical accountability in animal use, scientists can hardly hide behind an ideology that says that science is disconnected from ethics. And in the face of public law that requires that pain and suffering be controlled in animals, research workers cannot sustain ideological agnosticism and skepticism about animal consciousness.

Scientists are growing increasingly comfortable with talking about felt pain in animals as they respond to the law. Yet the ideology of science is still alive and well. The psychological community's response to USDA Animal and Plant Health Inspection Service (APHIS) requests for help in interpreting the Animal Welfare Act Amendments of 1985, mandating living environments for primates in research which "enhance their psychological well-being," has been, "There is no such thing." (The USDA tellingly replied, "There will be soon, whether you help us or not.")[23] The publication of *The Question of Animal Awareness*, which merely presented evidence for the modest proposal that animals are aware, elicited vituperative reviews from scientists rooted in the traditional ideology.[24]

The denial of consciousness persists strongly in animal science and animal agricultural research. Because food and fiber research is not covered by the federal laws mandating detection and control of research animal pain and suffering, animal agricultural research has been able, to a large extent, to maintain both physicalization of pain and stress and agnosticism about animal mentation. The animal science community has tended to see the long-term stress response as a nonspecific, "on or off" response. Until an important paper by Dantzer and Mormède published in 1983,[25] and even thereafter, animal science ignored pioneering work by Mason and others showing that the degree of the physiological stress response in a given case is under the control of and modulated by the animals' cognitive and emotional and thus mental states.

The common sense of science's claim that one cannot know animal mental experience is bad philosophy. The same positivism that would exclude talk of animal consciousness from science would also exclude talk of an external world that exists independently of perception, talk of minds in other human beings, and the knowability of the past. Evolutionary continuity and neurophysiological and behavioral analogies across species favor the claim that animals experience pain, and the fact that the failure to feel pain is biologically disastrous in human beings so born or suffering from such conditions as Hansen's disease is ample evidence that animals also feel pain and do not merely exhibit pain mechanisms and responses. In addition, although we cannot directly perceive thoughts and feeling in animals, we cannot directly perceive quanta and black holes either, or, for that matter, minds in other humans; all are postulated theoretical entities that are presumed to exist because they provide us with the best explanations for certain phenomena and enable us to predict features of those phenomena.

The key point for our purposes, however, is the incompatibility of the denial of animal consciousness and feeling with research into animal welfare, research demanded by the emerging social ethic we have detailed. Ordinary common sense now not only takes it for granted that animals can feel pain, distress, fear, anxiety, pleasure, boredom, happiness, and other morally relevant modalities of mentation; it now *cares* about that morally, and cares a great deal. Thus, any research undertaken as part of the attempt to meet social concern about farm animal welfare must accord not only with such social moral concerns but also with the ordinary commonsense view that animals can experience the morally relevant modalities of consciousness. Any attempt to deny this fundamental commonsense dictum is likely to destroy the credibility of research as a vehicle for finding solutions to social concerns about animal welfare. As both Ian Duncan and I have forcefully pointed out,[26] mental states and feelings are *everything* to welfare—even such physical interests as food and water are important essentially because their thwarting results in suffering (a state of consciousness).

For this reason, farm animal welfare research should not consist solely of the sorts of things traditionally done—measuring cortisol, counting stereotypies. The moral dimension of such research activities must be kept in mind as the end to which these tools are directed: increasing happiness, eliminating suffering. The public morality that is directing that there be such research must also shape it, so that the means do not become ends in themselves. Farm animal welfare research is not basic research; like AIDS research, it is inquiry directed toward solving real, pressing problems. In this case, it is the problem of how we alleviate the suffering of farm animals in confinement and other agricultural systems. It is not necessary, for example, to prove that branding hurts; research should be directed toward finding an alternative, not toward belaboring the obvious. Similarly, as mentioned earlier, it will not work to use research to "prove" that highly confined animals are happier—such an effort will simply impeach the credibility of research with the commonsensical general public in light of its ethical concerns.

I am not saying, of course, that there is no value to cortisol measurement or similar activities; the key point is that, in welfare research, they must be seen as evidentially related to how animals feel and how social morality demands that they feel. It is thus disappointing that few animal scientists have even read Marian Dawkins's seminal book, *Animal Suffering: The Science of Animal Welfare,* let alone taken its methodological approach seriously; it is, in essence, a treatise on how one uses scientific evidence to support the claim that an animal is suffering.

The interpretation of stereotypical behavior in farm animals illustrates our preceding discussion. Stereotypical behavior is repetitive, useless behavior that animals show in response to confined, isolated (for social animals), or deprived environments; examples are bar-biting in pigs and pacing or cribbing in stallions. While some animal behaviorists have taken stereotypies as evidence of suffering, others have argued that they are mechanisms of coping (e.g., to relieve boredom). Joseph Stookey has eloquently pointed out that even if the latter position is correct, we are still putting animals into pathological environments that force them to the limits of their coping skills, something that must be corrected.[27] Thus psychological theory tells us that children develop multiple personalities in order to cope with intolerable abuse. We surely do not find this situation acceptable because of such coping.

Stookey realizes that even if research were to indicate, say, by physiological measures, that animals were coping via their stereotypies, common sense and public morality would not countenance the systems that produced the stereotypies. Coping is one thing; coping at a level the social ethic sees as tolerable or justifiable is another. In other words, there is a full range of animal behavior that is consonant with coping and staying alive, even as there is a full range of human behavior consonant with survival under varying conditions. But just as public morality does not deem the entire spectrum of human coping behavior morally acceptable—eating out of garbage cans, drinking out of puddles, and sleeping on the street, for example—so it will not morally accept living conditions that inexorably generate bizarre, repetitive, purposeless, and sometimes self-destructive behavior in animals. Even if the scientific community has, with a few exceptions, ignored suffering growing out of boredom or loneliness, concentrating instead on the definition of welfare that stressed considerations consonant with production values, it does not follow that the new social concern about animals, and the concomitant broader definition of welfare, will allow farm animals to live impoverished lives in areas hitherto ignored by science and production.

## Can Animal Suffering Be Assessed Scientifically?

The most thoughtful challenge to scientific ideology's claim that one cannot study animal subjective experience is Marian Stamp

Dawkins's succinct 1980 discussion, *Animal Suffering: The Science of Animal Welfare,* which is a prolegomenon to precisely the sort of research, consonant with the social view of animal consciousness, that the issue demands. Although Dawkins is rooted in scientific ideology in her professed attempt to separate ethical questions from scientific ones, she is quite explicit in her claim that welfare includes mental as well as physical well-being.[28]

Dawkins's thesis is that the subjective experiences of animals can be a legitimate object of scientific study. Although there is, in her view, "no single method which, by itself, can tell us about the emotional experiences that animals might have,"[29] there is a set of diverse methods that collectively can give us a probabilistic picture of when and to what degree animals are suffering.

Dawkins surveyed and criticized several approaches.

1. *Looking at physical health.* Although no one would dispute that physical health is a necessary condition for well-being of animals, Dawkins argues that it is not sufficient. Animals can still suffer mentally, for example, from boredom.[30] Just as physically healthy humans can be suffering, so too can animals. On the other hand, if animals are unhealthy, they are almost certainly suffering.

2. *Looking at productivity.* Productivity may be relevant to welfare, in that productivity testifies that at least certain animal needs are being met. But because productivity is fundamentally an economic notion, it is conceptually and often actually present in the absence of animal well-being. Indeed, "productivity" is itself ambiguous. It may refer to the economic success of an operation as a whole or to the performance of an individual animal. In neither case does it ensure absence of suffering. As we saw earlier, profitable production systems may be the causes of certain production diseases. Many individuals may suffer and die, yet the operation as a whole may still be profitable; individual animals may "produce," for example, gain weight, in part because they are immobile, yet suffer because of the inability to move.

3. *Comparison with wild counterparts.* This measure has often been used to assess suffering of farm animals. Many animal advocates claim that life in the wild is better than life in confinement. In and of itself, Dawkins argues, such comparisons are not definitive. Life in the wild may be different from life in confinement, but it does not necessarily involve less suffering, by virtue of the presence, for example, of predators or diseases (e.g., parasites) in the wild, which are absent in confinement. The domestic animals may be quite far removed from their wild counterparts and thus perhaps better adapted to confinement. Finally, not being able to perform certain behaviors that wild counterparts perform, such as fighting, does not in itself prove that suffering occurs in farm animals. Presumably, the presence or absence of suffering arising out of having or thwarting behavior depends on the nature of the behavior in ques-

tion. Thus comparisons with wild relatives are best seen as flagging areas of concern that should be considered, not as definitive indicators of suffering.

4. *Looking at physiological measures.* Physiological changes—for example, long- and short-term stress responses—may or may not betoken suffering. Many beneficial and even pleasant activities occasion physiological stress responses (exercise, eating, and sexual behavior are examples), and animals devoid of stress also do not do well immunologically. We do not know where the happy medium lies. Furthermore, the stress response often is occasioned by attempts to measure it. In addition, the connection between what the animal experiences and its physiological responses is unclear.

5. *Looking at behavior.* According to Dawkins, it is difficult to equate abnormal behavior with suffering, since the very behavior in question may indicate that the animal has adapted to extreme circumstances. In general, as with physiological measures, Dawkins argues that we cannot confidently equate mental states with behavioral events. I do not find this argument persuasive. Instead, I agree with Stookey's argument cited earlier: If we are forcing animals to the extremes of their adaptive capacity by the systems in which we are raising them, we are doing something wrong.

6. *Animal choice.* We may get a prima facie picture of what sorts of conditions animals enjoy and prefer by "asking the animals," that is, by letting them choose—for example, between open conditions and confinement or between types of bedding. The problems with this approach is that animals do not necessarily choose what is best for them and that their choices change with experience, conditions, and other factors.

Although the earliest experiments involved simple choices, this methodology has been considerably refined since the 1970s. One can see how much the animals are willing to work (by operant conditioning, e.g., pressing a key) to achieve something they desire, what they are willing to give up, what noxious experiences they are willing to endure to achieve their preference, and the like. All this can tell us not only what the animals prefer but how much they care, or, to use Dawkins's economic analogy, how "elastic" or "inelastic" is their demand.[31]

7. *Anthropomorphic extrapolation.* Finally, we may extrapolate from our own experiences to those of other animals. The limitations of this approach are obvious: we are very different from animals and may mistakenly impose our preferences on them. Presumably, such extrapolations are best made regarding fundamental states all creatures share, such as physical pain, hunger, and thirst. At the opposite end, animal boredom may be quite different from human boredom.

To Dawkins's list one can add another method based in anthropomorphic extrapolation. This involves intentionally creating certain (presumed) experiences in animals (for example, fear), noting the animal's range of physiolog-

ical and behavioral responses, and then examining certain agricultural practices for these signs.[32] Such a method is, however, morally questionable if the
experience studied is noxious.

Although no one of these methods is infallible, Dawkins argues that research in accordance with all of them can generate reasonable judgments
about the likelihood of suffering. Her position is compatible with both common sense and society's new consensus ethic and bridges the concerns of social thought and the scientific community.

## What Sorts of Research Should Be Undertaken?

As indicated earlier, the ultimate goal of research is to help
the agricultural industry accommodate the emerging ethic for farm animals in
a way that both recognizes the economic realities constraining agriculture and
makes current animal agriculture significantly more animal-friendly. This
means that innovations oriented toward the well-being of animals must be
achievable in the current economic context, while making major progress toward accommodating the animals' natures, especially their psychological and
behavioral needs. It should also address the other sources of suffering we enumerated earlier: production diseases and lack of attention to individual animals. It is likely that such innovation will generate some additional costs to
producers, since modern intensive practices have essentially ignored these
concerns for half a century. Research should produce modifications in current
systems that not only appear effective but whose effect in improving welfare
and respecting animal nature can be demonstrated and validated according to
the sorts of criteria discussed above. Research activity should not simply
throw money at the problem; it should also be able to demonstrate that it results in measurable improvements, not merely cosmetic ones designed primarily to placate the public.

Obviously, research funds can be fruitfully expended in a variety of directions, detailed in the discussion of specific production systems in Part 2.
The possibilities range from attempting to find alternatives to such traditional
objectionable management practices as castration, dehorning, and hot-iron
branding, which have nothing to do with the advent of confinement agriculture; to improving handling of livestock, slaughter of animals, disease control,
and transport, all of which are presuppositional to any animal agriculture and
deal with areas that cause welfare problems *and* economic problems; to making intensive production systems more animal-friendly. Of these three categories, the final one is clearly the most difficult, as it requires vectoring in new
modes of thought into agricultural science, namely, concern about psychological well-being of animals, a hitherto neglected area.

In attempting to generate the gestalt shift required for effectively addressing the last category, researchers can be guided by major changes that have recently occurred in two other areas of animal use in response to social ethical demands: animal research and zoos. Changes in the latter have been dictated by a growing understanding of the ethic we have described above on the part of those who manage zoos. As one zookeeper told me, zoos can no longer be "prisons" where animals eat, sleep, and defecate. Society now insists that the animals be happy as well as alive, presenting zoos with much the same challenge as confinement agriculture, that is, making confinement systems animal-friendly and capable of accommodating animal natures.

A similar demand was imposed on biomedical research by the 1985 amendment to the Animal Welfare Act, which mandated environments for primates used in biomedical research which "enhanced the psychological well-being" of these animals. We have already noted the dissonance this demand created vis-à-vis scientific ideology; nonetheless, since federal law demanded such changes, scientists could not avoid engaging the issues.

Activities in both these fields can serve as a model for research into changing confinement agricultural systems for the benefit of animals. A significant literature exists in each of these areas. We have already mentioned the necessity of looking at research in other countries such as Sweden, Canada, Switzerland, or Britain, where social concern about farm animal welfare arose earlier and was, in some cases, accelerated by legislative mandate. Indeed, the Swedish law was explicitly guided by an ethic very like the one we have examined. A thorough review of the progress that has already been made will reduce the need for reinventing the wheel.

The work of zoologist Hal Markowitz, on behavioral enrichment for zoo animals and, to a lesser extent, for laboratory animals,[33] provides us with an exemplar of what can be learned from other fields and a model for research in improving agricultural confinement systems. Markowitz has created enriched environments for a wide variety of species, ranging from bears to apes to otters to servals to research primates, and his work has been modeled on a scientifically sound view of animals that is in perfect accord with today's social ethic.

The social ethic demands that our agricultural systems fit animal natures. Few thinking people, whether lay people or scientists, can deny that animals possess biological natures, which include a wide variety of physical and behavioral needs. In Markowitz's view, an animal is a bundle of *powers* that have been evolutionarily determined to fit a particular environment. The inability to use these powers, as occurs in confinement, generates frustration and incompatibility between animal and environment which is inimical to welfare.

Markowitz cites the case of servals, a South African feral cat, for which a new compound had been built at a zoo. The compound had been designed to replicate, as far as visitors were concerned, the indigenous environment for servals in the Kalahari Desert. The zoo had gone so far as to import native flora and rocks from South Africa. Nonetheless, the animals were listless and depressed, were not eating, and, in general, were languishing. The exhibit, which was meant to be a showpiece, attracted fewer and fewer visitors.

After studying the natural behavior of these cats in South Africa, Markowitz concluded that they had evolved for predation—specifically, for predation of low-flying birds. They would flatten themselves against the ground, await the overhead passage of birds, and leap into the air to catch their prey. Clearly, despite the fact that the zoo enclosure *visually* mimicked the Kalahari environment as far as human visitors were concerned, it did not at all *functionally* replicate the native environment as far as the animals' powers were concerned.

Markowitz then reasoned as follows: The key to a serval's telos was predation, yet one could hardly supply the animals with a steady stream of birds. Could one create a functionally equivalent environment in confinement that would allow the animals to exercise the powers constitutive of their natures and thereby alleviate their boredom and depression? It occurred to Markowitz that perhaps one could deliver the animals' food in some way other than simply giving it to them. He devised a compressed air cannon that sent meatballs sailing over the enclosure at random intervals throughout the day. Functionally, this replicated the prey the animals are built to capture.

The response was spectacular. The animals' behavior was transformed overnight from listlessness to electric excitement. Correlatively, the exhibit became the showpiece of the zoo, and visitors were enthralled by watching the animals express their natural behavior.

In my view, this case is a model of the sort of research that should be funded in response to the new social ethic's concerns about confinement agriculture. It is an excellent example of what needs to be done to satisfy public concern while adhering to economic constraints: making the animals happy in creative ways without wreaking economic havoc. This sort of applied research will probably produce the greatest return on money invested vis-à-vis satisfying social ethical concern about farm animal welfare.

## How, Morally, Ought Welfare Research Be Conducted?

Having discussed the ends of a research program relevant to social concern about the well-being of agricultural animals, we must now examine the means to achieving those ends. Society has expressed, in law, the rules by which medical research must be conducted. Central to these constraints is the demand that animal pain and suffering be controlled. According to the law, local committees of scientists and nonscientists review protocols and facilities to ensure compliance. Although the initial motivation was to control the use of animals in medical research, the law was rapidly extended to behavioral and wildlife research. Plainly, rationality dictates that an animal is an animal, regardless of the human use to which it happens to be put. If we as a society are morally concerned about the pain and suffering experienced by animals used in research, that concern cannot rationally be selective. If we want control of postsurgical pain in mice used in medical schools in cancer research, it is not rational to deny that same level of concern to mice used in private industry's cancer research or in agricultural research. Nonetheless, that is precisely the situation that currently obtains.

The two major pieces of legislation regarding the well-being of research animals, the 1985 amendment to the Animal Welfare Act and the NIH Reauthorization Act of 1985 (which turned hitherto unenforced NIH policy into law), cover many animals used in biomedical and behavioral research, but not all. Rats, mice, and birds have not, since its inception in 1966, been covered by the USDA/APHIS regulations interpreting the Animal Welfare Act, though, as we saw, a federal judge has ruled that failure to include them violates the legislative intent of the act. Though NIH policy does apply to these animals if they are used in NIH-funded research institutions, rats and mice used in private or corporate research contexts are currently covered by neither NIH policy nor the Animal Welfare Act. Many corporate research programs meet and even exceed the legislated requirements, but such compliance is voluntary.

More relevant to our purposes is the fact that farm animals used in agricultural (food and fiber) research are also unaffected by the Animal Welfare Act and NIH policy (the former statutorily exempts agricultural research from its purview). This situation gives rise to the following sort of fundamentally incoherent scenario, drawn from a real case I experienced.

Imagine a flock of sheep maintained for research at a university. The researcher in question uses the animals in both biomedical and agricultural research. Let us further imagine that one of the ewes gives birth to twin males. One of the lambs is fated to go into a biomedical research project, one into an agricultural project. Both require castration as part of the protocol. The lamb destined for biomedical research will be anesthetized, have surgery under aseptic conditions, be supervised during recovery, and receive postsurgical analgesia. The lamb entering the food and fiber protocol, in dramatic contrast, may be castrated with a pocketknife or have his testes bitten off by a shepherd, as often occurs under field conditions.

This is clearly absurd—so absurd that many animal care and use committees have demanded the same level of care for such procedures whenever they are performed and whatever the purpose. Such committees have also demanded anesthesia for invertebrates where it seems clear that a procedure is

likely to produce pain, despite the fact that the laws do not include invertebrates.

As Kant long ago pointed out, an overriding element of morality is con-
sistency. It is not a demand of benevolence but a fundamental component of
justice and fairness, and, indeed, of reason. Given that animals used in agricultural research and biomedical research are similar in all morally relevant
ways, they are entitled to similar treatment in all morally relevant situations.

It is sometimes argued that agricultural research animals are designed to
model animals that will be used in unregulated situations, as in the case of the
second lamb mentioned above, and thus should not be treated any better than
the animals they model. This argument is open to two responses. First, the fact
that pain and suffering is not controlled in farm animals is one of the fundamental reasons for and concerns of the new social ethic for animals. Thus, to
argue from what is done under field conditions to what should be done under
research conditions is to beg the question. One of the major motivations for
welfare research is to change field conditions so as to satisfy public concerns.

Indeed, as Hiram Kitchen, chairman of the AVMA Panel on Pain and
Suffering, a group convened to help explain the new research animal laws
with regard to the notion of pain and suffering to the research community,
pointed out to the panel, the law's demands for controlling pain and suffering
articulate the social standard for animal treatment. Thus the fact that agricultural practice deviates from these standards is not a justification for the status
quo; it is rather a mandate for agriculture to change its practice to be more in
accord with socially mandated standards![34]

Second, many features of research do not replicate the situations the research is intended to model. Rats are not people; cages are not the real world;
artificially high doses of toxicants do not reflect natural ingestion patterns;
cattle with rumenal fistulae differ from ordinary cattle. Research differs from
what it replicates in myriad ways. It could be argued that although providing
anesthesia for castration, for example, does indeed not replicate field conditions, it controls a variable, that is, pain and suffering induced by surgery,
which can affect what *is* being studied. As expressed in federal law, the social
ethic asserts that the only possible times pain and suffering should not be controlled in animal research of any kind is when it cannot be, that is, either when
pain and suffering are the direct objects of study or when one can demonstrate
that all possible methods for controlling pain and suffering will inexorably
skew what one is looking at in one's research and that the research is valuable.
(Sometimes control of pain and suffering skews the data in a way that can be
accounted for predictably.)

Furthermore, if the USDA, as the research arm of agriculture, is to take
the lead, through research, in responding to social concern about animal pain
and suffering in agriculture, it should respect these concerns in its own intra-

mural and extramural research programs. In this way, by taking the high ground, it will ensure credibility of its programs regarding animal welfare with the general public. Failure to do so is likely to generate public distrust regarding the seriousness and sincerity with which the USDA takes animal welfare and could precipitate loss of credibility in research as an answer to farm animal welfare concerns. This, in turn, could precipitate the passage of ill-considered legislation regarding agricultural research, agricultural production, or both. Agricultural research that will be undertaken to answer socioethical concerns about farm animal well-being should be like Caesar's wife—beyond reproach.

Thus, agricultural research should adopt something like the standards for animals used in biomedicine, at least as far as the control of pain and suffering is concerned, before the public becomes cognizant of the current double standard and agricultural research loses credibility. Facilities for housing agricultural animals used in food and fiber research should be clean, state-of-the-art, and well kept, but they do not need to meet the high standards demanded by biomedicine. They should, however, be animal-friendly, and such devices as metabolic stalls should be improved. It would behoove USDA to develop meaningful rules for agricultural research; the current guidelines essentially rubber-stamp the status quo. This is as much a prudent imperative to protect research as it is a moral imperative to protect the animals.

## Animal Welfare and Genetic Engineering

All future animal agriculture research should include in its planning the welfare concerns emerging from the new social ethic. Adherence to this point is especially relevant to genetic engineering of animals and their products. Thus far, both publicly and privately funded research in this field has been remarkably cavalier about public opinion in all areas, not just in the domain of animal welfare. The result has been a marked lack of social acceptance of genetic engineering and its products. Surveys repeatedly demonstrate the public's ambivalence about biotechnology, particularly the widespread concern that society in general has not been adequately consulted regarding regulation and release of biotechnology products.

The most obvious examples of this disregard of public opinion are the development of bovine somatotropin (BST) and the May 1992 FDA announcement that genetically engineered foods would undergo no special testing or labeling. Both these incidents bespeak the extent to which the government and private industry have radically omitted dealing with public concerns from their biotechnology agenda. In early 1993, the Campbell Soup Company disavowed the use of a genetically engineered tomato it spent millions to develop, because of fear of public rejection.

In the case of BST, were Jeremy Rifkin asked to orchestrate a scenario to give biotechnology a black eye, he could not have done better. Here was a product perceived by the public as tampering with milk, a foodstuff symbolizing purity and fed to children. Here was a product based in the use of a hormone (indeed, one of its names was bovine growth hormone) at a time when "hormone" is a scare word. Here was a product that would, in the public's mind, produce more milk when there is already a milk surplus and would, according to small dairy farmers, put them out of business. And to cap it all off, here is a product rumored to hurt the animals and developed by large chemical companies.

A similar degree of heedlessness was displayed by the FDA when it failed to specially test or label genetically engineered foodstuffs, apparently expecting consumers to be untroubled by, among other things, tomatoes containing flounder genes! I happened to be lecturing at the National Agricultural Biotechnology Conference in May 1992 at Texas A&M when the FDA made its announcement. The conference participants were so upset by the FDA's disregard of public sensibilities that, in a move I have never before witnessed at a scientific conference, they voted unanimously to ask their board of directors to send a strong letter of disapproval to the agency.

In my view, such disregard for public concerns foolishly and needlessly jeopardizes social acceptance of biotechnology. For a technology to win adherence from the public, it must be understood, not feared, and operate in accordance with prevalent social morality. If, as we have argued, a new (but essentially conservative) ethic for animal treatment is becoming operative in society, and that ethic demands that animals used for public benefit be happy (or at least not suffering), then genetic engineering of animals must respect that ethic. It should not engineer animals that will suffer by virtue of the engineered modifications. It should not engineer animals whose well-being is sacrificed to productivity, for example, oversized animals that experience foot, leg, and joint problems because of increased size. On the other hand, genetic engineering can contribute positively to farm animal welfare in many ways, for example, by enhancing disease resistance, as USDA researchers have already accomplished.

As I have suggested elsewhere,[35] genetic engineering of farm animals should be constrained by what I call the Principle of Conservation of Welfare, which asserts that animals should be no worse off by virtue of genetic engineering than they or the parent stock would have been without it. This principle can be useful in all animal production research, not just genetic engineering. Research should be the route to solving socioethical concerns about farm animal welfare, not a vehicle for creating new and additional welfare problems.

Of course, as the case of the so-called Beltsville pig (the oversized pig genetically engineered by introduction of the human growth hormone gene) demonstrates, we often cannot know the welfare results of genetic engineering until we perform it.[36] Therefore, we must do everything possible to diminish suffering of test animals—use the minimum number, control pain and suffering, and establish early end points for animals whose pain and suffering cannot be controlled. The classic "three R's" of W. M. S. Russell and R. L. Burch—reduction, replacement, and refinement—should be kept in mind as an ideal. With a proper research mindset, genetic engineering can provide a powerful tool for improving agricultural animal welfare. On the other hand, given intense public suspicion of transgenic work, researchers should err on the side of extreme caution, going out of their way not to produce either dangerous monsters or suffering monsters.

In view of the fact that the concern for animal welfare is not a fringe or passing fancy, and that research into farm animal welfare is a viable way to respond to public concern, it would be wise for USDA to undertake the following tasks immediately:

1. Survey European work in this field.

2. Survey U.S. agriculture for extant viable alternatives to problematic practices. (For example, many pork producers do not fully confine sows.)

3. Develop better methods for disseminating current knowledge pertaining to welfare—for example, principles of handling and transportation.

4. Appoint an advisory body of producers, scientists, welfare experts, and public members to construct general policy for funding welfare research and for ensuring that it addresses the issues.

5. Add a resident welfare ethologist to USDA's permanent staff.

6. Work quickly to make USDA's welfare requirements for agricultural animal research consonant with the ones that apply to biomedical animal research.

# PART 2

# Research Issues in Farm Animal Welfare

We have so far delineated the ethical and social basis for public concern about farm animal welfare. It is evident that, as far as mainstream thought is concerned, such concern is neither radical nor outrageous. While the public is not rejecting animal products, it does demand assurance that farm animals live happy lives under conditions that accord with their biological and psychological natures. This demand is consonant with what has already occurred in the area of animal use in biomedical research, where public law has articulated the call for control of animal pain, suffering, and distress in science. Despite the fact that some segments of the research community have opposed such controls, warning that they will impede research, jeopardize the discovery of cures for disease, and entail great costs, society has stood firm. The agricultural community should learn from the biomedical experience and engage farm animal welfare issues proactively. Since there have as yet been no sensationalistic incidents or press accounts to galvanize public demands for reform in confinement agriculture, the industry has an opportunity to demonstrate its concern for welfare issues.

The best form for such action to take is research into alternatives to agricultural practices that cause pain, suffering, distress, disease, or injury, in tandem with research into methods for

making confinement systems more animal-friendly, that is, more in accord
with the biological and psychological natures and needs of farm animals.
What areas of animal agriculture demand, and would benefit from, such research?

Unfortunately, there are few unbiased discussions of these questions in
the relevant literature. Industry representatives, naturally reluctant to give am-
munition to their critics, are loath to articulate forthrightly the problematic areas of their industry. Indeed, in many cases, industry representatives may
themselves have never thought through these areas. Thus, for example, I have
been told by beef specialists in animal science and by representatives of cattlemen's and cattle feeders' associations that, to their knowledge, there exists
no accurate survey of the welfare problems in the cattle industry. Critics, on
the other hand, tend to have only an outsider's view and are often misinformed. For these reasons, identifying the areas that need reform is not a simple matter. Furthermore, as noted in Part 1, what counts as a welfare issue
worthy of research or correction depends on the values held by the person
making the judgment. A producer will be inclined to worry about those issues
that affect productivity; an animal activist may see as problematic anything
that causes momentary pain.

My own strategy in identifying these issues involves several components.
In the first place, having taught a course in ethical issues in animal agriculture
for fourteen years, I have garnered a familiarity with most of the production
systems and have identified areas of concern regarding animal welfare. Further interactions with agriculture students, faculty (many of whom are themselves producers), and producers in the industry, all of whom enjoy a great
deal of expertise regarding these production systems, have refined my understanding of welfare concerns. In addition, my extensive interactions with people in the animal welfare community have given me a good sense of the sorts
of concerns they have (or would have) regarding animal agriculture.

In order to augment my knowledge, I have engaged in specific, extensive
discussions with producers, animal scientists, veterinarians, and welfare advocates on the matter at hand, namely, what welfare issues they see as requiring research effort. I consider those issues brought forth by all parties to the
debate to be most exigent and most likely to benefit from a significant research effort.

In schematic terms, I am seeking to identify the shaded area in the figure
on the next page. The unshaded areas represent mostly nonmainstream positions. For example, in the unshaded portion of the animal advocate circle, one
might find someone arguing that, since all animal use is immoral, we should
be spending research money on producing meat protein in fermentation vats
by biotechnology. On the other side, one might find a hard-core producer arguing that no welfare problems exist in current agricultural practices and,

therefore, no research money need be expended. We shall largely ignore such extreme positions, for reasons detailed in Part 1.

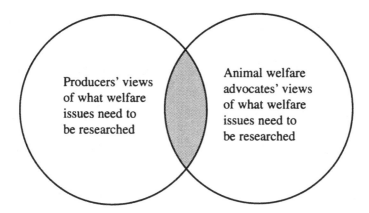

We are herein making the assumption that virtually all mainstream welfare concerns can be identified by this method. It is, for example, very unlikely that the public might have a concern not articulated by either animal advocates or producers. If such a concern did exist, it is probably based on misinformation and is not a research issue but rather an educational one. For instance, I once received a phone call asking me if certain animal producers did, in fact, severely beat their animals before slaughter, so as thereby to tenderize the meat!

Having indicated the basis for our delineation of welfare issues, we turn now to specific industries.

# 3 The Beef Industry

The beef industry has two distinct components, cattle ranching and cattle feeding, though it is often the case that the same individuals are involved in both sectors. Of all production systems, beef production most closely approximates the social ethic of husbandry. The ranching aspect of the industry, wherein animals live their lives under the conditions for which they were evolved, is virtually the same extensive system it was one hundred years ago, and feedlots are the least problematic of all intensive production units.

Despite this fact, beef has received a considerable drubbing in the press over issues of environmental despoliation, food safety, health, and animal welfare, most notably "downer" animals. The beef industry has been blamed for misuse of public lands, ozone depletion and the greenhouse effect, wasting of grain that could allegedly be fed to people, cardiovascular disease and cancer, and the exploitation of women.[1] Ranchers have been portrayed as eagle-shooting, environmentalist-lynching, plutocratic land barons, tooling around in Rolls-Royce pickups with steer horns on the front.

I have long argued the falsity of this stereotype. Many ranchers are small family farmers who must often work multiple jobs to hold on to their ranches. Furthermore, they are the standard bearers of the old husbandry ethic that society is trying to preserve—their animals are more than mere economic commodities to them. Few ranchers have ever seen their animals slaughtered; even fewer wish to. The vast majority see themselves as stewards of land and animals, as living a way of life as well as making a living. Many express significant distaste for industrialized agriculture.[2]

The beef industry could turn the animal welfare issue into a credit rather than a debit. Because ranch animals live their lives in accordance with their natures, and feedlots provide an environment that is not as radically removed from those natures as that of other confinement industries, beef could be marketed as the "ethical product" or "humane product" if certain practices were abolished or reformed. By and large, the welfare problems extant in the beef industry are either carried over from historical ranching by a combination of inertia and tradition or would be economically advantageous to fix, as well as welfare-advantageous. Although the beef industry at the feeder level displays some of the problems associated with industrialized agriculture, they are far less severe than those in poultry or swine production. Concerted research in some of these areas could produce quick and gratifying results.

## Welfare Issues in Ranching

As one might expect, given the traditional, extensive nature of cattle ranching, it has essentially no welfare problems growing out of the industrialization of agriculture. Many of the welfare problems in ranching are therefore of long duration and reflect solutions to management problems that have been sanctified by time, custom, and culture. This has militated against the search for alternatives and also works against ready acceptance of even economically advantageous solutions. Anyone dealing with cow-calf ranchers would do well to remember that the cow-calf aspect of the industry is as much a way of life as it is a business. Many ranchers work two or more jobs to sustain their way of life and resist any innovations that appear to them to compromise that way of life.

That is not to say that ranchers do not recognize the welfare problems associated with the cow-calf business. In my seminars to ranchers, I have little difficulty eliciting from them the triumvirate of branding, castration, and dehorning. Nor is there any attempt on their part to deny the pain and distress associated with these practices. On one occasion, while speaking to a large group of ranchers, I asked them to comment on the claim, common in scientific ideology (see Part 1), that the animals did not feel pain, or did not really feel pain, during these procedures, specifically focusing on castration. One rancher responded in a manner that drew cheers from his peers. Drawing his pocketknife, he asked me, "How'd you like *yours* cut off with this?" And on further questioning ranchers, I have invariably found them to be quite uncomfortable with causing pain to the animals. By and large, they see themselves as stewards of the animals. Thus, not surprisingly, many talk of nursing sick calves in their kitchens in a manner transcending cost-effectiveness. And again, few ranchers had ever been to a slaughterhouse, and virtually none wished to visit one. This ethic of stewardship disposes ranchers toward non-invasive alternatives that are cost-effective.

I recently found myself in the middle of a battle that graphically illustrates the courage, inherent decency, and concern for husbandry that characterizes western ranchers. In late 1993, USDA announced that it would be hot-iron face-branding an *M* on the jaws of all cattle entering the United States from Mexico. Such cattle importation had increased significantly with the advent of the North American Free Trade Agreement, and the USDA was concerned with clearly identifying Mexican cattle in case they were carriers of tuberculosis or brucellosis. Although the concern was legitimate, many people, myself included, were appalled by face-branding. After all, the face is highly innervated, for, from an evolutionary point of view, an animal would want to protect its facial region above all else, since the sense organs are located there. Thus the pain and fear associated with face-branding must be significantly worse than that of rump-branding—imagine, for a person, how much more a slap on the face hurts and distresses than a similar slap on the rump.

On learning of the announcement, I protested to some USDA officials and wrote a letter of concern along with A. P. Knight, a prominent cattle veterinarian and head of the Department of Clinical Sciences at the Colorado State University College of Veterinary Medicine. In the letter, Knight suggested ear-punching as a viable alternative to face-branding. Despite the fact that USDA had been convicted of violating animal cruelty laws in New York State by mandating face-branding in 1985, our protests were ignored. Some of my colleagues attempted to get the National Cattlemen's Association (NCA) to oppose the USDA policy, but it did not take a position. I then began calling individual ranchers whom I know personally, and all were appalled. Shortly thereafter, I was invited to a meeting of the Board of Directors of the Colorado Cattlemen's Association—all working ranchers, none bureaucrats—to explain the problem. Within a half hour of hearing the case, the board gave me an unequivocal statement: "As ranchers, we take pride in our long tradition of care and husbandry of our animals. While we realize that imported cattle may pose a health hazard to the domestic herd and must be permanently identified, we encourage USDA to adopt viable alternatives to jaw branding."

Taking this position was a courageous act, given the fact that the NCA opposed any action. As I left the meeting, I asked the board what I could do with the statement: Did they wish me to use it quietly with USDA? Could I publicize it? Could I share it with animal advocates fighting the USDA policy? I shall never forget the reply one man unhesitatingly offered: "Doc—we talked the talk; you walk the walk. It's your document, use it however you think best." This incident confirmed the view that I had already developed in many years of interaction with western ranchers—they are the finest, most decent, most honorable people I have ever known, and they care a great deal about their animals. Such people do not deserve the cheap shots taken at them by Jeremy Rifkin and others of that ilk.

On the other hand, the problematic practices of branding, castration, and dehorning are part of a rich cultural heritage going back four and more generations. Many brands, for example, have been passed on from father to son for well over one hundred years. Even Robert E. Taylor, a rancher and animal scientist who is the author of the excellent textbook *Beef Production and the Beef Industry: A Beef Producer's Perspective,* which stresses the need for business acumen in ranching, displays his own multigenerational family brands in a figure in the book, with evident pride.[3] So integral are the castration and branding of calves in the way of life that they represent a major family event, in some respects the most important coming-together of the year. One extension agent told me of a rancher whose sons, a physician and an attorney in California, come home to the ranch for castration and branding but rarely return for Christmas!

In this area of animal agriculture, then, as in no other, cultural components loom large and may be as important as economic factors; they must be kept in mind when alternatives are being researched and promulgated.

## Branding

The use of hot-iron branding as a management tool goes back 4,500 years to ancient Egypt; pictures from an Egyptian tomb plainly demonstrate the practice. Branding has two purposes. First, the hot-iron brand provides a form of permanent, unalterable identification, which enables the rancher to prove ownership and serves allegedly as an impediment to rustling. In many western states, brand laws, administered by politically powerful brand inspectors, mandate hot-iron branding as the only acceptable form of identification. Second, branding provides a readily identifiable mark for stockmen who are grazing their animals along with animals owned by other ranchers on open range. Any alternative to branding must perform these functions.

The animal welfare problem with branding is, of course, that it creates a third-degree burn on the animals. This burn is not only painful; it is a significant stressor that can cause weight loss, or shrink, due to animals going off feed. Furthermore, as ownership of animals is transferred, animals may be repeatedly branded—as many as four or more times. The cost to the livestock industry of branding is considerable; branding lowers the hide value for leather by some $7 per head, and the total annual cost to the industry is estimated to be $196,266,420.[4]

The most obvious alternative to branding is simply not branding. Branding does not, after all, protect against rustling; increasing numbers of rustlers are butchering cattle as they steal them, and the stolen animal is transported as boxed beef. In Colorado, there has been a rash of theft of dairy cattle, some at gunpoint. Nonetheless, branding is required by law in some states in order to sell cattle, and some readily visible, permanent identification system is seen as necessary by most ranchers.

The loss of hide value caused by branding provides an incentive to stop the practice. This incentive pertains to the final owner of the cattle, however, usually not the rancher, yet it is the rancher who has an interest in branding, for reasons discussed above. Were there a system whereby the rancher could receive at least some of the financial benefit of the unbranded leather, ranchers would have greater incentive to use other forms of identification, to petition for abolition of brand laws, or to develop new forms of identification. Research into the nature and viability of such an incentive system would help accelerate an end to hot-iron branding.

Other forms of identification, permanent and nonpermanent, are used to varying degrees in the cattle business. *Freeze branding,* now performed using an iron cooled with liquid nitrogen, is used on cattle and horses. Though freeze branding is certainly not painless, as some have suggested;[5] research indicates that it is probably not as painful as hot- iron branding.[6] We know from human cryosurgery that some pain is involved. Less tissue destruction occurs than with heat branding—only enough is required to destroy the melanocytes. No hide damage occurs, and the hair then grows out white permanently.

Despite these putative advantages, there are many disadvantages to freeze branding. Freeze branding requires more labor than hot-iron branding, more equipment, clipping the hair before the procedure, and a good deal of skill. Furthermore, it produces effective identification only on dark-colored animals, such as Angus, and is virtually useless for light-colored animals.

Another permanent form of identification, used primarily in purebred herds as a basis for identification and record keeping, is tattooing of the ears. The main disadvantages of this method are that it is very time-consuming and does not allow for visual identification from a distance.

Colored and numbered ear tags and neck chains meet the requirements of visibility but fail the test of permanence. Both can be lost by cattle, and neck chains present the additional problem of snagging and hurting or even choking the animals.

Much attention has been given of late to microchips that can be implanted subcutaneously with a hypodermic and read with a transponder. While meeting the criterion of permanence and unalterability, this technology fails on two grounds. First, the system is expensive: each chip costs about five dollars, and the transponder is very costly. Equally important, the transponder can read the chips only from a distance of no more than about five feet. So, though it is ideal for cattle in a chute, it does not help with visual identification under range conditions.

A promising method of permanent identification can be found in nose printing.[7] This approach takes advantage of the fact that each animal has a pattern of ridges and lines on its nose that, like a human fingerprint, is unique and unchanging throughout life. The procedure is simple, requiring only placement of the animal in a chute, a stamp pad on which to roll the nose, and a card on which to make the print. This process is fast, easy, and reliable but at present is used only on show animals. Nose printing meets the requirements of permanence and unalterability, ease of application, and economy. The print could be computer-scanned, digitized, and stored in a computer for easy record keeping and comparison.

The only drawback to nose printing is that, like microchips and tattoos, it does not allow for easy visual identification or any other identification at a distance. However, these methods could be supplemented by ear tags or by paint branding for sorting. Paint branding could be accomplished with a bright, indelible paint that could be applied to a shaved area each time the cattle were worked (most people work their cattle at least twice a year). This dual approach should be studied for viability—for example, to determine how long the paint remains visible. In general, all these approaches would benefit from simple and inexpensive research, ideally under ranch conditions at their most severe. I find nose printing most attractive; it is cheap and leaves no residue in the carcass.

Another approach is in its infancy. Joseph Stookey and his associates in Saskatoon have been experimenting with a compound that depigments hair permanently by acting on melanocytes. Stookey applies the compound to the animal in a brand pattern via hypodermic injection. The result is similar to freeze branding.[8] This type of approach should also be further studied.

Finally, some have suggested the use of genetic fingerprinting.[9] Genetic information on each animal could be obtained from blood samples and the information stored. The advantage of this over other approaches is that the information could identify not only stolen cattle but also meat from these animals if butchered. Such a method should be pursued, along with attempts to make it economically feasible.

## Castration

Castration represents another welfare problem, for it is accomplished with no anesthesia or analgesia. Castration is done both for tenderness of meat and for manageability of the animals, castrates being easier to handle than bulls. Calves are generally castrated when they are quite young, usually when they are branded, at anywhere from two weeks of age to two months, most often from six to nine weeks of age. In Britain, castration is not permitted after eight weeks of age unless anesthesia is used. In the United

States, some animals are not castrated until they reach the feedlot, when they may be eight or nine months old.

It is widely believed (as evidenced in the British law) that castration at a very young age results in a painless experience for the animal. (That thesis was, until recently, echoed in human medicine; open heart surgery, for example,was performed on neonates without anesthesia.) There are, however, no good grounds for believing that pain experience is tied to age.[10] It is well known that cattle are born precocious, and it would be biologically and evolutionarily incredible that all faculties are formed at birth except pain capacity. (People make precisely this claim, though—one veterinarian told me that pain-processing areas in calf brains are not fully myelinated until months after birth.) There are only two valid reasons for early castration: It is safer for the person doing the procedure, and controlling bleeding is easier since there is less vascularization and less testicular development at this age.

Although most range castration is done with a knife, there are a variety of other methods. None, however, is painless, and none can be viewed as an absolutely humane alternative to the knife. These methods include the use of Burdizzos, or emasculators, which are essentially pincers or pliers that crush or sever the spermatic cord and the blood vessels that supply the testicle. The lack of blood supply to the testicles leads to their deterioration. A similar mechanism underlies the use of the elastrator, which stretches a rubber ring over the testes, thereby shutting off blood supply and creating necrosis, eventuating in sloughing off of the testicles.

I have been told by some veterinarians that the Burdizzo approach is more humane than the knife in young animals because of the lack of blood supply. The claim is that little swelling occurs and the calves seem less agitated. On the other hand, we know that ischemia does result in pain. In older animals, the swelling is significant with both these "closed" methods. A comparative study of these methods in terms of pain signs and pain physiological parameters at various ages would be fairly easy to perform. It is unlikely, however, that any of these approaches would be fully acceptable to the new social ethic.

More acceptable to public ethical concerns would be anesthesia, local or general, for standard knife castration. This approach has been much discussed but little implemented, for a variety of reasons. Most important is the extra time associated with the process—waiting for a local anesthetic to take effect—which would decrease efficiency. This is even more true of general anesthesia, which would involve not only time but expense for the drug and risk to the animal. And even if anesthetics were used, the issue of postsurgical pain and its management remains. Development of an economically viable anesthetic (and analgesic?) protocol (almost certainly local) that could be used under range conditions efficiently is a viable research issue.

As mentioned earlier, animals are sometimes castrated at a relatively advanced age of seven or eight months. Temple Grandin has pointed out that about 50 percent of all calves from the Southeast are castrated when they arrive at the feedlot.[11] In such a case, anesthesia would be indicated for reasons of both animal and human safety. Nonetheless, such castration is often accomplished with restraint alone, for reasons of custom and expense. Xylazine, a plausible anesthetic for such a procedure, is expensive. Research into safe and cost-effective anesthetic regimens for such castrations would again be desirable. (Judging from my own experience with xylazine castration of eight-month-old bulls in a research project, I believe that the cost of the anesthetic is offset by the lack of complications of the sort that ensue in unanesthetized animals, but I cannot prove this.) Research into cost-effective anesthetic protocols is exigent.

The most rational and elegant solution to the issue of castration is simply not castrating. Bulls are much more efficient at converting feed than are castrates—this has been proved beyond a shadow of a doubt. Furthermore, bulls produce leaner meat, which is what fat-conscious consumers want. The industry unquestionably receives a double black eye because of castration. First, the public is angered over the animal welfare issue of surgery without anesthesia. Then, to replace the growth hormones supplied by the testes, the industry implants additional growth hormones in the ear. As one industry source said, "We take the testes off and put them in the ear." The public is frightened of "hormones in the food," and thus beef is criticized on food-safety grounds. Plus, the implants do not work as well as the testes!

For all these reasons, the industry would benefit from not castrating. In addition, the cattle can be marketed at 13 to 14 months of age, 3 months earlier than steers, at the same weight. Equally important, consumers cannot tell the difference between meat from young bulls (up to about 14 months) and steers.

Why, then, do cattlemen not raise bulls, as is done in Europe? There are a number of reasons, most of them nonrational. In the first place, the culture of the cattle business is strongly biased against raising bulls. Some ranchers assert that raising bulls is impossible, despite the fact that Europeans do it, that producers such as Martin Jorgenson have done it with "Dakota Lean," and that animal scientists such as Curtis Bailey have demonstrated its viability for years.

It is certainly true that one cannot manage bulls in the same way one manages steers, but young bulls are quite manageable. For example, bulls raised together can establish a dominance hierarchy to control fighting and, if kept together in feedlot pens, will not fight.

The more serious impediment to raising bulls stems from some nonrational marketing forces. At the moment, packers dock bull carcasses substantially, some one hundred and fifty dollars per carcass. There is no real justification for such docking: "They do it because they can," said one beef marketing expert. One story is that the public will not accept bull meat, but there is no evidence for this claim, since taste panels cannot discriminate between young bulls and steers and since the public is demanding the sort of leaner meat bulls produce. Of course, meat from five-year-old, three-thousand-pound range bulls is tough and unpalatable, but that is not what is being proposed. In any case, there is no requirement that bull beef be labeled as such at the retail level, though USDA graders label it "bullock," which in turn discounts the carcass.

There are some rational concerns about raising bulls. One is improper management, for if one attempts to export steer management systems unchanged to bulls, one is courting problems. Another is a higher percentage of "dark cutters" (undesirable darkening of the carcass) in bull carcasses, a function of stress, to which bulls are more susceptible than steers. Still another is the greater toughness of bull meat after 13 or 14 months, the optimal time for slaughter.

Raising and marketing bulls rather than castrates, as an answer to the castration issue as well as a way to increase efficiency, presents a series of research topics. The following areas are some that should be investigated:

1. Genetic changes in bulls to minimize stress susceptibility and dark cutters.
2. Management and handling techniques that minimize stress.
3. Genetic changes in bulls to maximize tenderness.
4. Simple, cost-effective management systems for raising bulls.
5. Consumer attitudes about bull meat.
6. Ways of changing the docking of bull meat by packers.
7. Changing the negative attitudes of producers regarding bull meat.

Such research has significant implications for the good of the industry beyond addressing the welfare issue.

Another possible alternative to castration is provided by immunological castration, which I have investigated in conjunction with the Colorado State University Department of Animal Science.[12] The approach is to conjugate LHRH (luteinizine hormone releasing hormone), or some other hormone responsible for the spermatogenic cascade, to a foreign protein. The conjugate is recognized as foreign by the animal's body, and antibodies are produced against it, thereby interrupting its effect. The conjugate is administered by injection. This approach has shown promise; in our own work, we found immunocastrates to be midway between castrates and bulls in growth, behavior, and other dimensions; their carcasses, when killed at about 13 months, were very palatable. On the other hand, their semen was still viable. One major impediment to this method, even if perfected, is the question of consumer acceptance. Would the male public accept meat treated with a demasculinizing compound? Research would be valuable to assess consumer acceptance. If consumer acceptance is not a problem, further research into perfecting the method could solve the welfare problem and benefit the industry, since immunocastrates are more efficient than steers.

## Dehorning

The presence of horns on commercial cattle is considered a problem because horns inevitably lead to damaged hides and bruising of cattle under range and feedlot conditions, especially during transportation. Cattle with horns also require more space in trucks and in feed bunks. Furthermore, some horned cattle become aggressive and bully other cattle away from feed and shelter. Though both horned and hornless cattle establish a dominance hierarchy, the problem is exacerbated by the presence of horns. Packers usually dock horned cattle.

Horns have been managed in a variety of ways, and it is obviously best to deal with them when the calf is young and the horn bud or button is very small. Probably the least invasive and traumatic method for removing horns is chemical, which should be done as early as possible in the calf's life. The caustic chemical, applied to the horn button, prevents further growth of the horn. Since the chemical is caustic, however, it can be irritating to the calves.

A second method, also feasible only when the calf is relatively young (under 5 months of age) is the use of a hot iron to burn the horn button. This procedure is not painless, since the interior of the horn is innervated.

A third strategy involves using devices such as the dehorning spoon or tube, which gouge or lever the horn out of the skull. The older the animal, the more developed the horn and the more traumatic the operation. In an animal that is relatively mature, such horn removal is, in the words of one veterinarian, "a bloody mess." When performed with clippers or saws, the procedure is again bloody and traumatic. Most dehorning is done by stockmen, not veterinarians, and local anesthesia is virtually never used, except by certain veterinarians who insist on it after a certain age in calves. Generally, the procedure is done under physical restraint.

Dehorning inevitably causes some pain and distress to the animals, ranging from irritation if chemicals are used to significant pain and trauma if mature animals are dehorned. Dehorning is sufficiently traumatic to have negative economic implications. A 1958 study from South Dakota showed that, when yearling steers were dehorned, two weeks were needed for them to catch up to their weight at dehorning; because of shrink arising from the trauma, the dehorned steers never caught up in weight to their horned counterparts.[13] The significance of this statistic was underlined by a 1968 study of more than half a million cattle in twenty-four states, which showed that the average age of cattle at the time of dehorning was 5.2 months, old enough for the procedure to be traumatic.[14]

The best solution to dehorning is the introduction of the poll (horn-free) gene into cattle, which eliminates the need for dehorning. Some of this work has already been done, but widespread acceptance has been slow, first of all because both bull and cow need to be homozygous for the poll trait to ensure that offspring will be polled. Since such matings are rare, people cannot depend on producing offspring and thus do not bother. Second, and more important, polled animals are widely perceived to be inferior in desirable traits to nonpolled animals, since they have not been subjected to the exhaustive breeding programs that have perfected horned cattle. One could, in principle, produce consistently superior polled cattle by an intensive breeding program aimed at that goal, but it would be quite expensive. A colleague of mine who is a dairy and reproduction specialist has estimated that introducing the polled gene and preserving other superior traits in Holsteins would raise the price of milk 4 to 5 percent.[15]

The most plausible approach to introducing the polled gene is probably genetic engineering. Such an effort is hampered by the fact that not enough is known about the polled gene. Here, then, are two research areas germane to cattle welfare in the beef and dairy industries. Research into optimal breeding of the polled gene could be undertaken. Similarly, government or industry could underwrite research into studying the mechanisms and effects of the polled gene, with an eye toward producing polled cattle transgenically. Such research would probably produce benefits in other areas of the cattle business as well, since the first transgenic calf was produced only in 1993 at Colorado State University. The gene for double-muscling was successfully introduced, but untoward results occurred—the calf was unable to stand up on its own a few weeks after birth.[16] This case illustrates poignantly the possible negative welfare effects of inserting genes before their mechanisms and actions are fully understood.

Though branding, castration, and dehorning are second nature to the cattle business, they are not essential and may even in some cases (e.g., branding) be counter to economic rationality. Animal welfare is an excellent catalyst for challenging these management techniques. When I talk to ranchers, I ask them to engage in a thought experiment: If tomorrow the law banned branding, castration, and dehorning, would they go out of business? Their answer is, "Of course not!"

## Cancer Eye

Both state cattlemen's associations and the NCA have identified cattle with ocular neoplasia as a major welfare concern. White-face cattle, especially Herefords, are highly susceptible to the development of ocular cancer, known in the vernacular as "cancer eye." Advanced stages of cancer eye are painful to the animal—indeed, pain specialists have identified ocular pain as one of the most extreme and disturbing forms of pain. In addition, cancer-eye animals create, as it were, a "black eye" for the industry, projecting to consumers an image of unsafe food. According to the January 1992 report of the Animal Care Work Group of the NCA, "the condition [of cancer eye] should not be allowed to progress beyond a treatable stage before marketing."[17]

As the NCA report indicates, this problem raises some research issues. The report recommends that a chart be developed to depict the various stages of cancer eye and the proper treatment at each stage. Development of this chart should be the responsibility of the USDA's Food Safety and Inspection Service. Research into the dangers for the food supply associated with cancer-eye carcasses would also be desirable[18]—condemnation now occurs in a fairly imprecise way, based on gross observations of lesions. Existing research has characterized the genetic tendencies toward cancer eye; additional research into the molecular genetic basis of cancer eye and into transgenic strategies for replacing the defective gene would be very useful.

## Cattle Handling

The handling of cattle at all levels of the industry, from cow-calf to slaughter, has major implications both for animal welfare and for profit. Poor handling can result in significant stress, pain, and injury, leading to animal suffering and distress and to loss of income from bruising, greater susceptibility to disease by way of immunosuppression, increase in prevalence of dark cutters, and lower reproductive rates.

Several historical reasons exist for poor handling. One is cultural—there is a long precedent of "cowboying" the animals among some ranchers, though most producers know that "gentling" is best. Such rough and rowdy handling, roping, and wrestling of animals is, for some ranch workers, the very soul of working cattle. One expert in ranch management told me of a consulting job he had done for a large Montana ranch, where he was asked to observe ranch activities and make recommendations for cutting costs and making operations more efficient. At the end of two weeks of scrutiny, the consultant called in the ranch owner and told him that the largest single source of inefficiency was cowboying the animals. For example, in roping a sick or injured calf, one should strive for gentleness and minimal excitement, yet some ranch hands did precisely the opposite, riding hell-for-leather and roping the animal at high speed. "Hell," replied the owner, "if I couldn't cowboy the animals, I wouldn't want to be in the business."[19]

Thus, part of poor handling is attitudinal. This macho, domination attitude can be found throughout animal agriculture and, in the cattle business, in feedlots, salebarns, cattle transport, and packing houses, not only in cow-calf operations. Finding effective ways to change that attitude represents a valuable research question, as gentleness is often equated with lack of masculinity. For example, in salebarns, one frequently sees employees—cowboy "wannabes"—beating and prodding animals unnecessarily with hotshots.

A second source of poor handling is lack of knowledge of cattle behavior. Many people in the cattle business have no idea of flight distance, balance point, reasons for balking or stampeding, and other fundaments of animal behavior. Only two individuals, Temple Grandin and Bud Williams, have focused on using behavior to aid handling. Effective methods for imparting available information to those handling cattle should be studied, and research should further continue into cattle behavior.

A third source of poor handling is poor equipment or improper use of extant equipment. Poor equipment is often attributable to a lack of knowledge of animal behavior—for example, many loading chutes are designed in a manner counterproductive to their purpose. Some equipment may have sharp edges or hazards that bruise or startle the animals. Research into animal-friendly equipment should be a major priority. Many animals are injured, traumatized, or "spoiled" by improperly designed, used, or maintained squeeze chutes.[20] Restraint devices not requiring handling to catch animals running through a chute should be researched, as should animals' responses to restraint. It has been reported, for example, that sight restriction reduces stress of restraint, and such ethological principles should be employed in studies regarding animal handling.[21] Temple Grandin's conveyor restraint system and L. M. Panepinto's sling restraint device for hogs are examples of animal-friendly restraint systems.[22] Grandin has pointed out that "development of improved restraining devices is hampered by a severe lack of funding. Construction of working prototypes is costly, and the industry has been unwilling to provide funding."[23] Such an area would thus benefit from government research or funding.

## Transportation

The transportation of livestock represents another prime concern, from both a welfare perspective and an economic one. Transportation has been a major problem to the industry since the turn of the century, when the Livestock Conservation Institute was founded to diminish the significant losses incurred by the industry. The losses stemming from transportation—bruising, injured backs, dark cutters, shipping fever, and other stress-related diseases—are enormous, as high as 25 percent.[24] Bruising alone cost the industry $22 million annually.[25] Unfortunately, relatively little progress in improving transportation of livestock has been made, and the costs in welfare are on a par with the economic ones.

The welfare problems associated with transportation pervade the entire process. Loading and unloading are often accomplished with unnecessary roughness, hotshotting, and ballyhoo, which is frightening and stressful to the animals and can cause bruising. The actual transit conditions can expose the animals to extremes of temperature, depending on the season. The ride is generally rough, especially on rural roads, subjecting the animals to loss of balance, bruising, stress, shrink, difficulty of subsequent weight gain, and fear. Most of the animals are unaccustomed to being transported, and the very novelty of the experience is a significant stressor, especially in light of evidence that novelty of environment is more stressful to cattle than electric shock.[26] It is not uncommon to see animals on a higher truck deck defecating and urinating on lower animals. Not only is this probably a stressor, since animals tend to avoid one another's excrement; it is a mobile advertisement against the beef industry. I recall my son, at age six, viewing such a scene with horror and saying, "That's not right!"—surely a universal reaction.

There are many research issues in this area.

1. The degree of stress (objective) and distress (subjective) experienced by transported cattle, using the criteria delineated in Part 1.

2. Ways of making the ride smoother and more comfortable. Grandin has argued, for example, that air ride suspensions, used on semitrailers that transport fragile goods, could be far less prone to traumatize animals than conventional suspensions.[27]

3. Ways to detect and alleviate other noxious aspects of the ride, such as wind sway.

4. The question of ideal trailer design, taking into account the animals' needs and natures. This includes research into flooring that reduces slippage.

5. The effects of extremes of climate during transportation and how to mitigate them.

6. The effects of dust, exhaust, air circulation or lack thereof, carbon monoxide, and even length of exhaust pipe, along with ways of minimizing their negative impact.[28]

7. The effects of noise and how to reduce it.

8. Protocols for ideal management of animals on long hauls, including feed and water regimens, time on truck, ideal procedures for on- and off-loading, and whether rest stops should be mandated.

9. Cost-effective methods for preconditioning or training animals to truck rides. Some cattlemen have developed ways of preconditioning or "backgrounding" cattle for transportation. Some of these methods have been successful, some not; all are costly and labor-intensive. Work by John Archer

and others has shown that stress (and distress) responses are mitigated by familiarity.[29]

10. Ways to reduce transportation and auction time. The less transportation and the less exposure to unfamiliar circumstances, the better for the animals. Often cattle are sent through many auction markets before they reach the feedlot, with each market stop constituting a new stressor. Limiting such stops is better for the animals, and a law to that effect, allowing calves to be sold at only one auction, would be useful. Research into use of videotapes and live television marketing should be emphasized. At present, such marketing is not practical for small groups of cattle.

## Downer Cattle

The marketing of sick, crippled, or "downer," nonambulatory cattle is a major welfare problem in the cattle business. The television coverage of the treatment of such animals at the Minneapolis–South St. Paul stockyards in 1990 elicited strong negative responses from the public, as well as proposed legislation against the practices. There are few sights more outrageous than watching a crippled or downer animal being dragged off a truck by a tractor. Indeed, such dragging of a conscious animal is already illegal at USDA-inspected packing plants, according to the regulations promulgated under the Humane Methods of Slaughter Act of 1978. However, the law does not cover livestock markets, farms, feedlots, ranches, or dairies.[30]

Downer animals should be moved on some mechanical conveyance when they arrive at their destination. Many downer animals are cows culled from dairies. Others are sick or injured animals who have not received or responded to medical treatment, or emaciated animals. Still others are male Holstein calves newly born. Producers should be fined for shipping such animals, as is done in portions of Canada. As one rancher told me, "We should eat our mistakes." Suffering animals should be euthanized immediately at the farm, or, if they have gone down during transport, as soon as they arrive at their destination.

Though downers are a major industry problem, so recognized by the NCA[31], they do not in themselves represent a subject for scientific research. The issue is one of management and regulation.

## Slaughter

The most pressing problems associated with slaughter grow out of the absence of preslaughter stunning in Muslim (halal) and kosher (schechita) slaughter. In both these areas, stunning is forbidden by current interpretation of religious law. Despite the fact that some countries ban such slaughter, it persists in the United States.

The first point that must be settled in discussing this issue is an empirical one: is the ritual slaughter in question indeed inhumane? Work by C. C. Daly and colleagues on cattle, published in 1988[32], showed a significant difference in time to loss of visual and somatosensory evoked response and loss of spontaneous cortical activity between animals that were stunned and those that were killed by throat-cutting in ritual slaughter. In animals stunned by captive-bolt, the loss of evoked response was immediate and irreversible. Loss of spontaneous cortical activity occurred in under 10 seconds. In the nonstunned cattle, evoked potentials were lost between 20 and 126 seconds after cutting, with a mean of 77 seconds for somatosensory responses and a mean of 55 seconds for visual responses. Spontaneous cortical activity was lost between 19 and 113 seconds (mean, 75 seconds) after cutting. The time difference was smaller in non-stunned sheep, which lost consciousness within 2 to 15 seconds.[33] The difference between species is probably a function of differing anatomy in cerebral blood supply.

All this seems to indicate that what is plain to common sense is correct: being stunned is preferable to not being stunned. (We are here assuming that consciousness during bleeding out is not pleasant.) In New Zealand, Moslem slaughter is forbidden without stunning. Significantly, some Moslem authorities there have permitted either mild mechanical stunning or electrical stunning of the brain.

Adding insult to injury, some kosher slaughter plants continue to shackle and hoist conscious animals for efficiency in processing, despite the fact that such activity seems to violate both the letter and spirit of the religious law underlying kosher slaughter.[34]

What are the research issues connected to these practices that seem to compromise animal welfare? In the case of the lack of stunning, it appears that among Moslems at least, there is room for modernizing slaughter. This possibility should be investigated with Moslem authorities in the United States. The Jewish situation is more difficult, as the tradition allows virtually no room for change. Thus, effecting the adoption of some form of stunning with Jewish religious authorities is unlikely.

On the issue of shackling and hoisting, alternatives do exist, specifically, the so-called ASPCA slaughter pen. Unlike the Weinberg pen, used in Europe, which turns the animal upside-down for slaughter, the ASPCA pen allows the animal to remain upright with the chin lifted up for easy slaughter. Research indicates that the animals prefer upright restraint.[35] Grandin has described using the ASPCA restraint pen, together with sharp knives and proper cuts, as a way of minimizing animal distress in kosher slaughter and accelerating loss of consciousness.[36] However, the argument that shackling and hoisting is still more efficient has held back adoption of more humane alternatives.

Research assessing alternatives to hoisting and shackling from a humane as well as an efficiency perspective should be undertaken. Ideally, the humane alternative should be compatible with efficiency. Failure to effect change in shackling and hoisting could well result in change by legislative mandate.

## Gomer Bulls

Ranchers need to know when cows are in heat. Because bulls have an obvious vested interest in heat detection, using them to detect heat is a time-honored approach. In order to keep the detector bulls from impregnating the heat cows, the bulls are surgically altered in a variety of ways.[37] The penis may be redirected to one side, creating so-called sidewinders. The penis may be amputated, retracted and fixed, or surgically adhered to the lower abdominal wall. Fistulation of the preputial cavity following closure of the preputial orifice, installation of mechanical preputial blocking devices, and the placement of an artificial thrombus in the corpus cavernosum penis are also used. When the altered bull mounts the cow, a marking device hung from his chin marks the cow in heat. All these methods produce some pain and much distress growing out of frustration, though the methods that redirect the position of the penis still allow the animal to ejaculate as a consequence of frottage. American men, when informed of these sorts of alterations, see them as the worst possible abuse.

There are alternatives for detecting heat that do not cause welfare problems, such as patches that are applied to cows, visual inspection, and use of cows or steers given testosterone, but most cattle owners believe bulls are the least fallible. Vasectomizing or epididymectomizing bulls would allow the animals to detect heat without being frustrated, and this has been done. The drawback is that there is considerable transmission of venereal disease and a high rate of endometritis in cows that have coitus with such bulls. The perfecting of a humane, effective, foolproof, simple heat-detection method or a method for eliminating the problems with sterile bulls is therefore an important issue for welfare research.

## Feedlot Problems

In the feeder portion of the industry, many of the problems mentioned earlier can surface in an amplified way. Late castration, branding, and dehorning of animals in the feedlot create major welfare issues, as well as economic setbacks. Proper handling and equipment is also a relevant concern.

There are also welfare problems unique to feedlots. One major issue is feedlot design. Poorly designed drainage systems compromise both welfare and productivity. Relatively little easily accessible information is available on designing and managing feed yards to accommodate young bulls. Design of chutes, ramps, and loading docks can be improved. (Almost all the work in this area has been done by Temple Grandin.) Research into elimination of liver abscesses caused by feeding "hot," high-concentrate, low-roughage diets would benefit both animals and producers. Closer attention to the health of individual animals would improve both welfare and economic returns.

Feedlots are the most animal-friendly of confinement systems, since they allow the animals significant room to move as well as social opportunities. Research could make them more animal-friendly. Shelter from wind, dust, sun, and snow would benefit animals and producers, as would sprinkling to cool animals and keep down dust. Research into ways of meeting some of the animals' other needs, especially behavioral ones, should be undertaken—for example, routine provision of scratching posts has always seemed to me an obvious improvement that would increase welfare at a low cost. I believe that a relatively small expenditure of research money could go a long way toward making feedlots the exemplary intensive system: animal-friendly, ethologically sound, yet embodying the advantages of environmental control to animal welfare.

# 4 The Swine Industry

Historically, the pig was the first farm mammal to be subjected to extremely intensive housing and management, a trend that has greatly accelerated.[1] Over 90 percent of pigs are raised in some kind of confinement.[2] At the same time, swine are almost universally considered the most intelligent of farm animals, possessed of a good deal of curiosity, learning ability, and a complex behavioral repertoire, and are thus "easily bored," as Ronald Kilgour puts it.[3] The complexity of pig behavior raises a host of issues relevant to rearing these animals under austere confinement conditions. Such conditions give rise to a significant range of behavioral anomalies in confined pigs, referred to in the industry as "vices." As Andrew Fraser and D. M. Broom[4] and I have pointed out, such a locution is misleading and downright inaccurate, for it suggests that the pigs are somehow to blame for the aberrant behavior they display under confinement conditions. The animals' behavioral anomalies result from an attempt to cope with conditions that frustrate their natures, or telos. Kilgour and Dalton note in their *Livestock Behavior: A Practical Guide,* "Pigs are easily bored and housing and management should be planned to provide for their inquisitive nature. This will prevent most vices, which are the result of boredom."[5]

Thus in the swine industry, unlike the beef industry, one encounters a host of welfare problems that are the direct results of the industrialization of agriculture and are based on thwarting the animals' behavioral and psychological needs and natures. As we saw, these sorts of concerns do not figure significantly in the beef industry, since the animals live most of their lives under extensive conditions and since feedlots do not violate the animals' natures to the extent that confinement swine operations do. Further, cattle are undoubtedly less intelligent and behaviorally complex than swine. It has also been suggested that cattle, being ruminants, have a source of stimulation (cud chewing) that monogastrics such as swine lack. Since the major problems in the swine industry grow out of housing conditions that, while congenial to economic efficiency, are fundamentally at odds with the animals' natures, some of the welfare problems associated with confinement raising of swine will be more difficult to resolve than welfare problems in the cattle business.

In general, the behavior of domestic swine is not far removed from that of their wild counterparts.[6] Many cases are known in the United States of groups of domestic pigs that became feral populations and displayed the entire behavioral repertoire shown by wild swine that were never domesticated. Moreover, controlled studies show that pigs born and reared in confinement, descended from generations of other confinement-born and -reared animals, will display "natural" pig behavior when placed in extensive conditions—for example, will head directly for a mudhole and wallow.[7] The most exhaustive study in this area was performed at Edinburgh University in the early 1980s by Alex Stolba and D. G. M. Wood-Gush, who placed domestic pigs in a "pig park," essentially a large enclosure replicating conditions under which wild swine live.[8] On the basis of such work, and other research into swine preference, one can get a sense of the full range of pig behavior and begin to understand the most serious areas of deprivation in confinement.

Although frustration of natural behavior is the most dramatic and problematic aspect of swine production, there is also a range of welfare problems related to management, disease, and transport which must be addressed.

## Swine Behavior

A summary of "natural" swine behavior and preferences can serve as a guide to identifying problematic areas in the confinement agricultural rearing of swine. As mentioned, Stolba and Wood-Gush studied pig behavior under open conditions in a "park" consisting of a pine copse, gorse bushes, a stream, and a swampy wallow.[9] Small populations of pigs, consisting of a boar, four adult females, a subadult male and female, and young up to about 13 weeks of age, were studied over three years. The researchers observed not only the behavior patterns of the animals but also how the pigs used the environment in carrying out their behavior.

It was found that pigs built a series of communal nests in a cooperative way. These nests displayed certain common features, including walls to protect the animals against prevailing winds and a wide view that allowed the pigs to see what was approaching. These nests were far from the feeding sites. Before retiring to the nest, the animals brought additional nesting material for the walls and rearranged the nest.

On arising in the morning, the animals walked at least 7 meters before urinating and defecating.[10] Defecation occurred on paths so that excreta ran between bushes. Pigs learned to mark trees in allelomimetic fashion. The pigs formed complex social bonds between certain animals, and new animals introduced to the area took a long time to be assimilated. Some formed special relationships—for example, a pair of sows would join together for several days after farrowing, and forage and sleep together. Members of a litter of the same sex tended to stay together and to pay attention to one another's exploratory behavior. Young males also attended to the behavior of older males. Juveniles of both sexes exhibited manipulative play. In autumn, 51 percent of the day was devoted to rooting.[11]

Pregnant sows would choose a nest site several hours before giving birth, a significant distance from the communal nest (6 kilometers in one case).[12] Nests were built, sometimes even with log walls. The sow would not allow other pigs to intrude for several days but might eventually allow another sow with a litter, with which she had previously established a bond, to share the nest, though no cross-suckling was ever noted. Piglets began exploring the environment at about 5 days of age and weaned themselves at somewhere between 12 and 15 weeks. Sows came into estrus and conceived while lactating.

One of Wood-Gush's comments is telling: "Generally the behavior of ... pigs, born and reared in an intensive system, once they had the appropriate environment, resembled that of the European wild boar."[13] In other words, there is good reason to believe that domestic swine are not far removed from their nondomestic counterparts. Thus, comparison of behavioral possibilities in confinement with those in the rich, open environment that pigs have evolved to cope with seems a reasonable way at least to begin to assess the welfare adequacy of confinement systems. If confined environments generate behavioral disorders in the animals, this represents additional reason to believe that there are problems with these environments. In the language of Part 1, we are in a good position to measure current systems against all aspects of the swine telos, physical and behavioral.

## Confinement of Sows

Virtually every expert with whom I have discussed the swine industry sees the confinement of dry sows as its major welfare problem. This view is echoed in books and articles dealing with swine welfare. These experts perceive the confinement of sows as problematic in two ways. First of all, it is truly a welfare problem. Plainly, many of the needs of the animals are not met in austere confinement systems. To be sure, as Colin Whittemore points out, confinement is not the only issue: "We are not suggesting excessively restrained pigs are happy—undue restraint is an important loss of welfare. But [our] work shows that restraint is not the only thing. By all means, let the pigs out, but don't think that solves all the welfare problems."[14] Whittemore is certainly correct; we shall shortly detail numerous other welfare problems in the swine industry, some of which are synergistically connected with sow confinement. But the second sense in which sow stalls are highly problematic is equally important. As we said in Part 1, the emerging social ethic for animals, and the attitudes connected with that ethic, will simply not accept sow stalling, regardless of scientific evidence. Joseph Stookey has stated this point beautifully:

> Such issues as sow stalls are destined to be resolved by moving in the direction towards systems which the public finds acceptable. Obviously the public is concerned about restricting the freedom of movement of animals and the public would prefer that such systems (such as tethers and sow stalls) be abolished. This is a response that has nothing to do with "welfare" from the pig's perspective (though they would argue that is the very essence of their concern)—they simply find stalls offensive from their own personal perspective and would like to see them abolished. No amount of scientific evidence would ever convince the public that such systems are not cruel.[15]

This statement is exceptionable in two ways. First, we have argued that "cruelty" is not the issue. Second, I believe that the notion that the public response has "nothing to do with 'welfare' from the pig's perspective" is overstated. Nonetheless, Stookey points up the indisputable fact that public perception should be of fundamental moment to the future of the industry. As agriculturalists often remark, "perception is reality." Stookey continues:

> If ... sow stalls continue to ... [be] an acceptable practice in the swine industry, I believe the days are still numbered before the public outcry will take over the legislation and force the government to ban the stalls. In the long run, the industry could be worse off and may lose credibility by not moving in a direction that satisfies the public.[16]

It seems clear that research issues associated with confinement of sows should enjoy top priority in the area of swine welfare. What, then, are these issues?

In the United States, sows are typically not tethered as they are in Europe. Instead, they are kept in gestation stalls while they are pregnant, for the vast majority of their productive lives, three to five years. The stall is approximately 2 feet wide, 7 feet long, and 3.3 feet high.[17] This extreme confinement allows a great many sows to be housed in an environmentally controlled situation, fed and cared for by a minimal and unskilled labor force, and maintained with minimal feed, for energy is not wasted on thermoregulation or movement. Such a system allows maximal production efficiency. It further allows people who may not be "pig smart," as one expert puts it, to work in a facility where the system compensates for lack of stockmanship. On the other hand, management makes the difference between a viable confinement system and a total mess.

Unquestionably, such systems have produced large volumes of pork at reasonable prices. And as confinement managers argue, there are certainly benefits to the animals. In parts of the country where there are extremes of temperature—for example, Colorado and the Midwest, where temperatures may range from –20° F to +100° F in the course of the year, and rain, snow, and wind can make life miserable—an environmentally controlled habitat set for the animals' comfort zone can be a boon. In addition, individual, as opposed to group, housing of sows cuts down on fighting and biting and thus on wounds and competition for food.

Nevertheless, the costs to the animal in terms of its telos is considerable, especially in the face of what we know of swine behavior under the extensive conditions in which pigs have evolved. Most obvious to the agriculturally naive observer, perhaps, is the lack of exercise. As I have pointed out elsewhere,[18] one need not be Konrad Lorenz to realize that all animals who have evolved with bones and muscles need the opportunity to use them. As seen in our capsule discussion of swine behavior, pigs under extensive conditions spend a good deal of time moving about. If a system does not allow such an animal even the room to turn around, it is reasonable to view it as thwarting some very fundamental needs or tendencies, needs that have both a physical and a cognitive component, thus leading to negative welfare. Animals that like to move and are built to move are surely affected negatively if they cannot do so.

Closely connected with the inability to move is the element of monotony, lack of stimulation, or, as Kilgour forthrightly put it, boredom.[19] Given the complexity of behavior and intelligence natural to the sow, the absence of possibilities in the gestation stall, and the emergence of stereotypies, it defies good sense to suppose that the animal is *not* bored. And I frankly do not cavil at the use of a word like "boredom," which the scientific ideology has shunned as "anthropomorphic," as we saw in Part 1. First, as even the popular press reports, anthropomorphic attributions are currently much in vogue in science.[20] Second, as an elegant article by Françoise Wemelsfelder has detailed at great length, one can provide precise, scientific meaning to terms such as "boredom" applied to animals.[21] Third, and most important, the common sense that informs social ethics will never doubt that sows are capable of being bored and will judge the system accordingly.[22]

A series of research issues emerges from the discussion to this point. One could, as has often been done, generate research to show that the animals adjust to lack of exercise and a deprived environment and that stereotypical behavior shows that they are coping. Such a tack would, I believe, be a serious error. The U.S. public will surely demand, as the European public has demanded, that the problems of boredom and exercise be addressed and that current systems be corrected in this regard. The research money is much better spent addressing these problems than attempting to assure the public that they are not legitimate concerns.

Three sorts of research strategies would be fruitful areas for research expenditure regarding the fundamental issues of movement, exercise, and boredom in sow management: modification of existing systems, development of new systems, and study of traditional systems. They are not mutually exclusive and in my view should all be pursued, at least to some extent.

## Modification of Existing Systems

For the short run, modification is certainly the most plausible approach. Can one change existing confinement systems so as to make them more animal-friendly with respect to boredom and exercise? This is a welfare research issue of paramount importance.

In what ways could modification be accomplished? The Moorman Manufacturing Company has provided an excellent example with its Moor Comfort system. Here the sow stall occupies the same area as conventional gestation crates, but the sides of the stall are hinged so that the sow can borrow space from the neighboring sow in order to turn around, groom herself, move, and so on. Research into costs, problems, and benefits of this system should be undertaken. Does it reduce stereotypies? Do the animals show a preference for the system? Does it satisfy or help satisfy public concern? Can the system be further developed to enhance the environment, for example, by provision of toys, straw, or varied diet? (Many farmers have provided bowling balls, tires, chains, and the like to confined pigs for some years to alleviate boredom, but that is not feasible in current gestation stalls for reasons of space.)

Another approach occurred to me as I viewed a large, full confinement system. Why not develop something analogous to pet doors that allow the animals to back out into an outdoor space at will? Such a space could be a large common area surrounding the building or individual outdoor runs (like dog kennels) with straw, the possibility of rooting, or other stimuli. All the sows or only a few sows could share a run; each sow could return only to her own run by computer coding, as in some existing pig and dairy systems. Such a system could alleviate boredom, lack of social contact, and lack of exercise.

Clearly, this approach raises many research questions. What would be the cost of modifying current facilities? (Probably minimal, I would guess.) How much extra feed would be required? Would the animals stay in during bad weather? (I suspect this would almost certainly be the case.) How much would they go out? Would stereotypies diminish? What other problems would arise? How much fighting would occur? How would disease and parasite control be affected? How would the runs be cleaned? What sort of flooring should the runs have? (Dirt? Sand?) How would the public see such modifications relative to improved welfare? How far would such changes go in mitigating public concern?

Another possibility, which should be looked at in tandem with any modification of stalls is the provision of straw.[23] Extensive evidence indicates that from the point of view of the animal, straw is highly desirable. It is used for nest building, bedding, and comfort; feed can be scattered into it to allow for foraging and rooting; and it can provide a dietary supplement. Indeed, straw seems to be a godsend to improve welfare of confined sows.

It has been suggested that diet for sows is closely involved with a tissue of welfare concerns, including boredom, which is why I raise it here. Sows in confinement are generally fed a measured ration of nutritionally balanced feed aimed at maintaining the animal for production. The animal eats it quickly, it is the same every day, and it does not necessarily provide a sense of satiety. As we saw earlier, pigs in the wild spend much time foraging. In addition, the natural diet is high-roughage; the confined diet, high-concentrate. Thus, while feeding of confined sows meets nutritional needs, it does not allow the exercise, stimulation, variety, and activity that foraging achieves. *Ad libitum* feeding has been shown virtually to eliminate stereotypies. This, together with our knowledge of swine behavior, tells us that preoccupation with food is a major part of the swine telos. Thus, if something could be done to address the inadequacies of daily feeding, it could make the animals much happier in confinement.

Straw is a plausible vehicle for alleviating this problem. Many of the standard stereotypies are food-related, or at least related to oral gratification.[24] Bar-chewing, chain-chewing, and vacuum (purposeless) chewing are relevant examples. Provision of straw to sows reduces or eliminates such stereotypies.[25] Furthermore, sows will eat the straw, an activity that not only reduces stereotypies and gives the animals something to do related to eating but also perhaps provides a feeling of satiety. For this reason, straw may well be a significant welfare advance for stalled sows.

The main reason straw is not given is that it interferes with waste disposal. Most confinement swine facilities use concrete slatted floors for waste disposal into manure-handling systems, and straw impedes their functioning. Additionally, straw is not as cheap as it once was and is labor-intensive to replace.

Herein lies a fruitful set of research issues: Given that straw provision reduces problems associated with boredom, frustration of eating behavior, lack of satiety, stereotypies, frustration of nesting behavior, and lack of bedding, leading to bruises and abrasions, is there a way that its use can be made compatible with current systems? What will it cost? How can it be reconciled with waste management?

## Development of New Systems

A long-term option for resolving the welfare problems associated with sow stalls is redesigning swine operations. Obviously, no industry is wedded to one way of doing things—buildings, capital investments, and machinery all become obsolete and require replacement. In my view, the industry would do well to start thinking about future systems that are both highly efficient and respect the animals' natures. Could such systems be as efficient as current systems in strictly economic terms? No one knows. Certainly that is a significant research issue. I believe we could come closer to current levels of efficiency than many producers suspect if we start rethinking our confinement systems now, and if improved animal welfare and efficiency are stipulated as givens for the future. In any case, this sort of planning is necessary to avoid having systems abolished (and/or mandated) by legislation based more on emotion than on careful reflection.

Are there guides to follow in developing such systems? Obviously, yes. Profitable semi-intensive and extensive systems exist that can help guide the industry (discussed in the next section). Hal Markowitz's approach to zoos (described in Part 1)—creating systems that allow the animals to express their natures, keep them from being bored and frustrated, and yet are essentially intensive situations that are in relevant ways *functionally* analogous to extensive ones—also provides a useful model. Research should be undertaken to try to exploit these ideas in the swine industry.

Another practical approach involves detailed and careful study of the European experience. Nearly all of Europe has felt strong pressure against confined sow systems, and in certain countries, Sweden being the paradigm case, their abolition has been legally mandated. How are these countries responding to these challenges? Indeed, most of the countries have put a good deal of money into farm animal ethology for a long time, in contradistinction to the United States. Knowledge of European thinking and action is appallingly scanty and sketchy in the United States, even among academics. (I have scoured departments of animal science and producer organizations for individuals and/or material with detailed information on the European reforms, with frustrating results.) Common sense dictates that we at least learn from European mistakes and not reinvent the wheel.

When I first undertook to prepare a report on farm animal welfare for the USDA, I stressed my desire to study European agricultural systems. I was dismayed to learn that I could not undertake travel to Europe on project money. This policy seems paradigmatically absurd—penny-wise and pound-foolish. A detailed review of European approaches could save enormous amounts of time and money and generate fruitful collaborative efforts.

### The Edinburgh Housing System

Fortunately, some information regarding alternative systems has consistently trickled in from Great Britain. A particularly interesting approach has emanated from Edinburgh. Wood-Gush and Stolba, who described swine behavior in their "pig parks," developed an alternative design for swine facilities based on their ethological studies. First described by Stolba in 1981,[26] this system continues to be refined at Edinburgh.[27] The basis of the system, a group housing approach, is the family.

Stolba's insight was similar to that of Markowitz—one can respect the telos of swine without fully replicating the extensive natural environment. After studying swine behavior in essentially natural conditions, as described above, Stolba went one step further and observed the behavior of similar groups of pigs in small paddocks with and without certain environmental features, such as bushes. He found that when the environmental features were present, the animals in the small paddock behaved virtually identically to swine under natural conditions. In the absence of what may be called the enriching environmental features, however, the behavior was changed. Out of this insight came the Edinburgh housing system (Figure 4.1).

Wood-Gush summarizes the system:

Stolba's research suggested to him that reduced space is not an impediment to maintaining behavior; it is the environmental features which contain the key stimuli and releasers for many of the behavior patterns that are important. He therefore designed a housing system containing as many of the key features which he could identify, placing them in the same sort of spatial relationship as outside. Briefly these included:

1. A sleeping area well away from the feeding area, as had been found in the semi-natural area.
2. Open-fronted pens to resemble the forest border habitat.
3. A dunging corridor to resemble the paths between bushes.
4. A rooting area, since about 51 percent of the pigs' time was spent in rooting.
5. An activity area that contained a marking post and bedding material to be collected by the animals.

The close social bonds of the animals were not forgotten in the design, for the basic unit of the system is a group of four sows well known to each other. Each has a pen and all four pens are connected by the dunging corridor. Each pen has a sleeping area which can be shut off and used as a farrowing pen with farrowing rails. Furthermore, from the sleeping area the pigs have a good sight line as in the outdoor nests, and

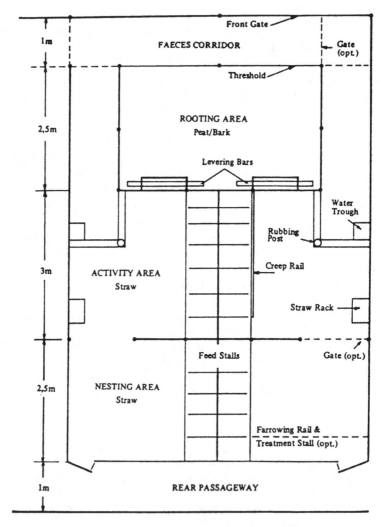

**Figure 4.1.** Edinburgh swine housing system: Stolba's ground plan and furniture for the enriched pen. The plan shows two pens of a unit of four pens for a family group. From Alex Stolba, "A family system of pig housing," in *Alternatives to Intensive Husbandry Systems* (UFAW, 1981), p. 56.

next to it is the activity area and outermost, the rooting area. Piglets born in the pen are kept there until the point of sale so that no other housing is required. Under these conditions the females tend to show synchrony of oestrus. The boar is brought in at 20 days after parturition and stays until all the females have been mated. By the time the next litters are born, most of the previous litters are ready for sale or have been sold.[28]

Colin Whittemore described subsequent work with this concept and the problems that arose.[29] The setup, depicted in Figure 4.2, is essentially the same as Stolba's. As before, four sows lived together; the boar stayed with them for 4 to 5 weeks. Weaning occurred naturally. All the animals lived together until the pigs were slaughtered at 5 months of age, 2 weeks before the sow farrowed again.

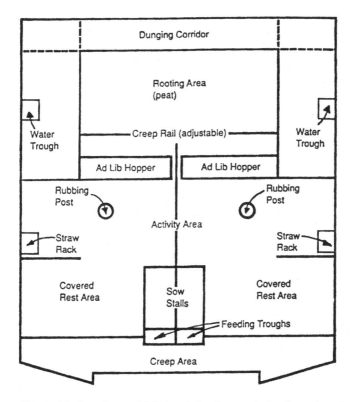

**Figure 4.2.** Experimental Edinburgh family pen design for swine. From C. Clanton, "Animal Welfare: Lessons from Europe," *National Hog Farmer,* Dec. 15, 1990, p. 62.

As the diagram illustrates, the pen was divided into a nesting area, rooting area, activity area, creep area, and dunging area. Environmental enrichers included rubbing posts, a straw rack, water and feed troughs, and *ad libitum* feeders for young pigs.

Whittemore lists some of the problems encountered in the facility.[30] They included the need for individual feeding of sows; otherwise the big ones got bigger, and the small ones got smaller. The dunging corridor did not work—the animals defecated all over the facility. The pen was very cold. The lack of farrowing restraint and cold led to 25 percent piglet mortality. But, said Whittemore, "from other aspects, the welfare is really very high. We solved the welfare problems of post-weaning stress, slatted floors, flat decks, and overcrowding at a stroke. If we can make the thing warmer and better controlled for the baby pigs, it can be effective."[31]

Obviously, the problems raised by Whittemore are candidates for research and should be investigated. Many other research questions are engendered by this system: What are its total space requirements and how would they affect construction costs? Table 4.1 shows Stolba's data on space requirements for intensive, conventional, and his family systems. How do pigs perform in this system? What are the feed-conversion differences in this system versus other systems? (According to Stolba, "for growing pigs, food input and conversion seems to be similar to conventional systems.")[32] Is the system economically viable? If so, could one persuade producers to convert to it? Would legislation be required or could a system of tax incentives help speed adoption?

Wood-Gush has raised another valuable point relevant to research questions:

> Although this system is still in the prototype stage, it does provide a very good example of how a sound study of the behavior of the animal can aid us in designing better housing. Closer investigation of the key stimuli guiding the main behavior patterns would be of value, for it might allow greater control and use of space. Ultimately knowledge of these stimuli should enable us to trick the animal into being able to perform those behavioral patterns of importance to it, and for us to guide it successfully away from behavior which we do not want, without causing frustration. Clearly, a knowledge and appreciation of the evolution of our agricultural animals together with information about the behavior of feral populations will aid us in assessing housing systems and welfare.[33]

For our purposes, this system provides some important lessons for the future, not only via-à-vis pigs but applicable to all research issues in farm animal welfare, especially those pertaining to confinement:

**Table 4.1.   Space requirements per sow for intensive, conventional, and enriched housing systems**

| | Pen measures | | | | | | Space allotted per sow or 10 fatteners[b] (m²) | Occupied per cycle of 166 days[a] (days) | Space required per sow and cycle | | |
| | Width feeding space (m) | Depth total (m) | Depth components (external) | | | | | | Intensive system (m²) | Conventional system (m²) | Enriched family system (m²) |
| | | | Dung area (m) | Lying area (m) | Trough (m) | ½ passageway (m) | | | | | |
|---|---|---|---|---|---|---|---|---|---|---|---|
| Pregnant (dry) sow | 0.65 | 3.60 | 0.80 | 1.90 | 0.40 | 0.50 | 2.34 | 124 | 1.75 | 1.75 | |
| Lactating sow and litter | 2.00 | 3.55 | | 2.10 | 0.70[c] | 0.75 | 7.10 | 32 | 1.37[d] | 1.37 | |
| Multisuck, sow and litter | 3.00 | 7.50 | 2.80 | 7.00 | | 0.50 | 22.50 × 1/3[e] | 15.4 | 0.54 | 0.70[f] | |
| Sows grouped for service | 0.50 | 5.40 | | 2.80 | 2.10[g] | 0.50 | 2.70 | 33.3 | 0.78 | 0.54 | |
| Boar and service pen | 5.40 | 2.90 | | 2.40 | | 0.50 | 15.66 | 1/20 per sow | 0.31 | 0.78 | |
| Grouped replacements[h] | 0.50 | 5.40 | | 2.80 | 2.10 | 0.50 | 2.70 | 47.3 | 1.16 | 0.31 | |
| Early weaning flatdeck[i] | 1.05 | 3.20 | | 2.50 | 0.70 | | 3.36 | 57.2 | | 2.64 | |
| Weaner pool (3 litters)[j] | 3.00 | 7.50 | | 7.00 | | 0.50 | 22.50 × 1/3[i] | 58.3 | | | |
| Total for breeding | | | | | | | | | 5.91 | 8.09 | |
| Growing fatteners[j] | 0.27 | 3.00 | 0.60 | 1.50 | 0.40 | 0.50 | 8.10 | 58.3 | 2.85 | | |
| Finishing fatteners[k] | 0.33 | 3.50 | 0.80 | 1.80 | 0.40 | 0.50 | 11.60 | 107.8 | 7.54 | | |
| Open-front fatteners[l] | 3.00 | 7.50 | | 7.00 | | 0.50 | 18.50 | 162.8 | | 18.40 | |
| Total for fattening | | | | | | | | | 10.39 | 18.40 | |
| Inclusive pen space | | | | | | | | | 16.3 | 26.5 | 28.5 |
| Space inside buildings | | | | | | | | | 16.3 | 26.5 | 25.5 |

Source: Alex Stolba, "A Family System of Pig Housing," in *Alternatives to Intensive Husbandry Systems* (Potters Bar, England: UFAW, 1981), p. 66. Reprinted with permission.

Notes: [a]Breeding performances calculated to be 2.2 liters/year, with 10 piglets/litter. [b]3 days for cleaning plus 10% safety margin. [c]Front passageway included. [d]3 weeks weaning. [e]5 weeks weaning. [f]5 sows/pen. [g]Individual feeding stalls. [h]0.4 sows per cycle to be replaced. Sows not conceiving culled 35 days after weaning. [i]Piglets up to 25 kg. Juveniles 25 to 50 kg. [j]Juveniles 25 to 50 kg. [k]Juveniles 50 to 100 kg. [l]Juveniles 25 to 100 kg.

1. Basic ethological understanding of the animals in question is vital. Such research should be undertaken for all farm animals in confinement.

2. The notion of melding such knowledge with practical constraints in the manner of Stolba and Markowitz is a very promising research strategy.

3. The idea of ongoing research into a welfare problem at a particular institution (Edinburgh, in the case above) is very attractive.

### Other Alternatives to Sow Confinement

In March 1993, I visited a large swine operation in Colorado that has been in existence since the early 1970s and is consistently profitable. The owner was very generous in spending time with me and devoted a good deal of attention to explaining his approach to swine-rearing. He does not, however, wish to be identified here, as he does not want to spend a great deal of time fielding queries, although he would be willing to share his approach and experience with researchers.

The operation has approximately 1,600 sows and covers about 40 acres. It is best described as semiconfinement. Boars are kept in individual stalls, and groups of pigs are finished together in finishing pens in an "all in, all out" way. The primary unique feature of this operation is the absence of gestation stalls. The sows do spend about four weeks in farrowing crates, to avoid crushing of piglets. But the rest of the time, they are not stalled. They are either grouped together in pens or kept outside. The pens are divided into two parts: a concrete portion and a sand portion. The pigs dig, root, and play in the sand; one sees virtually no stereotypical behavior in these animals. Fighting is not a problem either.

The outside pens appear to be, as it were, hog heaven. Some sixteen sows are kept in a large outdoor enclosure (about 40 feet × 100 feet), with a quonset shelter and some shaded areas. There is also a pool and a muddy area, and the animals are provided with straw. One gets a strong sense (admittedly subjective) that the sows are content and come far closer to actualizing their natures than they do in full confinement. Aggressive interactions among sows are not a problem, for they rapidly develop a pecking order.

The owner admits that he might do slightly better economically if he kept his sows in confinement. However, he and his manager of twenty years both feel that it is immoral to keep the sows in stalls. As the manager put it, "An animal that can't even turn around can't be happy or even comfortable."

The owner has experimented with finishing animals outdoors. He has found that the cost per pound of pork is two cents higher than when he finishes them indoors. When I asked him if he thought indoor feeding with the option of access to the outdoors might be more viable, he agreed that this is very possible and could and should be researched. He also felt that individual indoor housing of boars was not ideal from a welfare point of view and agreed that outdoor approaches should be investigated.

I came away with the strong feeling that his system was a viable, non-radical approach to many of the sow welfare problems, and told him so. He agreed in principle but added an important caveat. To make his system economically viable, he said, one needed first-rate labor and management, people who were "pig smart." In other words, the labor force must be knowledgeable about and sensitive to the animals. A full confinement system is far more "idiot-proof" and to be profitable does not require a high-quality labor force. His employees do not turn over often and are loyal to him and to the animals. He felt that many full-confinement operations are more bottom-line businesses than husbandry systems and that his system could therefore not be readily exported to such operations.

I strongly recommend that this operation be studied as a workable alternative to sow confinement, in view of the fact that the owner has been financially successful for more than twenty years. He felt that his system could be used successfully in all parts of the country.

In September 1990, the University of Minnesota Extension Service held a swine conference for veterinarians. In its published proceedings was a brief paper somewhat misleadingly entitled "Extensive Methods of Swine Production".[34] In reality, only one alternative system is described. Nonetheless, it is relevant to finding researchable alternatives to sow confinement.

The authors were concerned about the alarming rate at which small swine operations were disappearing and being replaced by confinement operations requiring high-energy input and high capitalization. With an eye toward this issue as well as toward "social issues regarding animal welfare" and "minimum stress as conducive to overall better performance,"[35] the authors studied a small group of twenty sows housed in an alternative system and compared it in a variety of ways to a similar group raised in confinement.

Although no detailed description of the alternative system is provided, the authors listed the following features: pen gestation, skip feeding during gestation, superinsulated waterers to prevent freezing without high-energy inputs, straw bedding, pen farrowing with removable cubicles, *ad libitum* feed consumption during lactation, a creep area for the piglets, and weaning at 4 to 6 weeks of age. The two groups had similar genetics and received comparable management and nutrition. The groups were studied for 18 months (i.e., three litters) and were compared in terms of productivity, economics, and behavior of sows and piglets.

In terms of productivity, the alternative group showed higher preweaning mortality and a lower number of pigs per sow. But sow condition was better and piglet weight higher at 3 to 4 weeks in this group.

In terms of economics, the differences are summarized in Tables 4.2 and 4.3. Average cost of facilities/sow place was 50 percent higher for the con-

Table 4.2. **Average monthly operating and overhead costs for alternative and conventional sow housing systems, June–December 1989**

| Item | Alternative ($) | Conventional ($) |
|---|---|---|
| Feed | 475 | 538 |
| Veterinary services | 82 | 96 |
| Straw | 20 | ... |
| Gas and electricity | 1 | 112 |
| Machinery | 47 | 18 |
| Taxes | 28 | 31 |
| Other | 13 | 36 |
| Total | 666 | 831 |

*Source:* C. Pijoan, P. E. Arellano, et al., "Extensive Methods of Swine Production," in *Minnesota Swine Conference for Veterinarians* (College of Veterinary Medicine, University of Minnesota, 1990). Reprinted with permission.

Table 4.3. **Labor requirements in alternative and conventional sow housing systems, June–December 1989**

| Activity | Alternative | | Conventional | |
|---|---|---|---|---|
| | Hours | % | Hours | % |
| Feeding | 60 | 19 | 101 | 27 |
| Cleaning | 50 | 16 | 75 | 21 |
| Moving pigs | 38 | 12 | 31 | 9 |
| Observing | 34 | 11 | 17 | 5 |
| Planning | 34 | 11 | 32 | 9 |
| Breeding | 21 | 17 | 20 | 5 |
| Other | 77 | 25 | 91 | 25 |
| Total | 314 | 100 | 367 | 100 |

*Source:* See Table 4.2.

ventional system ($800 vs. $1,200).

In terms of behavior, higher numbers of stereotypical behaviors were observed in the conventional group. In the alternative group, higher aggressive/submissive behaviors were observed only during the first half hour after the sows were fed.

These results, though only preliminary, provide yet another basis for research into an alternative system. It would be necessary to study how the lower capital costs and lower labor costs of the alternative balance out relative to the lower productivity. One would also need to know in detail what problems had arisen; what modifications, if any, could be made to reduce preweaning piglet mortality; how large the facilities were; and so on.

Other outdoor alternative systems are being researched at the University of Illinois College of Veterinary Medicine's Outdoor Pork Production Unit at Dixon Springs Agricultural Center and at Texas Tech University. A brochure from the Illinois group describes its system as follows:

The Production Unit is designed to provide pastures and equipment to far-row a group of six sows each week and husband their offspring to market weight. The unit is divided into gestation-farrow, nursery, and grow-finish subunits. The system was established to provide an outdoor production laboratory where intensified production procedures currently utilized in total confinement systems could be adapted to pasture production. All subunits were constructed on well-sodded fescue pastures.

It would be reasonable for the USDA to collect all the data from such experiments, synthesize it, and direct further research toward problematical areas.

A further alternative system is the Hurnik-Morris (H-M) system, developed by J. F. Hurnik and J. R. Morris (Figure 4.3).[36] This system, like that of Stolba, is based on careful ethological knowledge of swine behavior. It is a pen system, each pen housing six sows. The system allows "socially coordinated eating and resting, controlled and socially undisturbed feed consumption, physical exercise, and regular exposure to boars."[37]

Although economic comparisons between the H-M system and conventional ones have yet to be made,[38] there are production advantages to the sys-

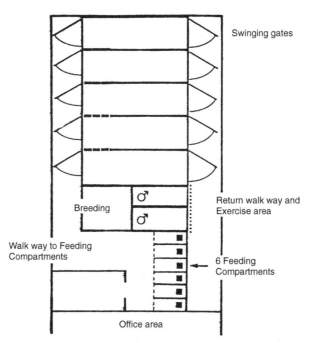

**Figure 4.3.** H-M swine housing system. From J. R. Morris and J. F. Hurnik, "An alternative housing system for sows," in *Canadian Journal of Animal Science* 70 (1990): 957 ff.

Table 4.4.    Farrowing performance of primiparous sows reared in conventional and H-M housing systems during gestation

|  | Conventional individual stall | H-M system |
|---|---|---|
| Number of sows | 25 | 22 |
| Pigs born/litter | 9.2 | 9.0 |
| Pigs born alive/litter | 8.6 | 8.3 |
| Pigs weaned/litter | 6.7 | 7.7 |
| Litter weaning weight (kg) | 50.0 | 56.9 |
| Piglet mortality (%) | 19.8 | 7.5 |
| Piglets crushed (%) | 11.8 | 3.8 |

Source: J. M. Morris and J. F. Hurnik, "Sows Housed for Freedom," *Pig International,* April 1991, pp. 11-13. Reprinted with permission.

tem, as shown in Table 4.4. This system should be studied further.

## Looking at Traditional Systems

The final approach to the welfare problems of sow confinement is probably the simplest: it involves looking at traditional systems of swine-rearing that did not involve total confinement. Many people still make a living raising swine under nonconfinement conditions. Paradigmatic examples of this approach can be found in the Midwest, where, for a variety of reasons, farmers have resisted full intensification. Many such farmers have survived economically and weathered drops in the pork market while others who went fully intensive lost their farms. It is easy to see why. A traditional pig production system involves raising pigs basically in the open, with inexpensive housing available for shelter during inclement weather. When the pork market is problematic, such producers simply get out of pork and put the land to other uses. The confinement farmer, on the other hand, must continue to make huge payments on expensive buildings and equipment and thus is likely to go under, unless the operation is part of a large corporate structure with vast resources enabling it to weather the economic storm.

In February 1993, one variation on such a traditional approach was described in detail by a swine veterinarian, George Bergman, working in Cass County, Michigan, which has the largest concentration of outside farrow-to-finish swine in the world.[39] The average operation contains five hundred sows and raises small grains, corn, soybeans, wheat, oats, and milo in addition to pigs. It uses small quonset-type shelters to house the animals, covered by one sheet of plywood in spring, summer, and fall and two in winter. Pigs farrowed in the spring are finished in the fields where they were born. Pigs farrowed in fall or winter may be moved to semi-intensive smaller lots with quonset hut protection.

The system is made possible by the soil and terrain. The land consists of rolling hills with a sand and gravel subsoil with rapid percolation. Thus the pig lots stay dry, and both the parasite load and number of enteric pathogens are kept down.

Standard wisdom says, as the veterinarian in the article puts it, "that parasites are impossible to control when pigs are on dirt." In his view, however, "they're not that difficult to control if you have a comprehensive program,"[40] which he proceeds to describe.

Successful outdoor farrowing requires lot rotation to minimize parasite and pathogen buildup. Although more feed is needed to maintain thermoregulation, that cost is counterbalanced by much less capital investment. According to Bergman:

> The fixed costs are less than they would be with conventional farrowing houses. Producers frequently run ten sows and their litters per acre—both spring and fall. Some of our medium-sized producers are now farrowing outside every month of the year. This provides a more constant cash flow whether they finish them all or sell some as feeder pigs.[41]

Unless pig farms are truly isolated from one another, disease control can be more of a problem outdoors. Reproductively, however, "producers typically wean litters of 7.5–8.5 pigs. That's within a pig or two a year of those farrowed in confinement and for considerably less in fixed expenses."[42]

All aspects of this system should be looked at, particularly with regard to viability in other portions of the country. How, for example, would this system fare in warmer climates or in areas with different, less ideal, soil types?

## Farrowing Crates

Farrowing crates were devised to prevent sows from crushing piglets, a common phenomenon under extensive conditions. Generally, a sow spends about a month in a farrowing crate, from directly before parturition until weaning of the piglets. Since the point of farrowing crates is to restrict the movement of sows so they cannot turn around, and since the farrowing crates are about the same size as gestation stalls, the same welfare problems relating to restricted movement we have discussed vis-à-vis gestation stalls arise here. Farrowing crates have also been correlated with some pig diseases, including dystocia, agalactia, and wasting disease.[43]

Because farrowing crates demonstrably provide a way for diminishing crushing of piglets, they could perhaps be justified to the social ethic if the sow were not confined at other times. For example, in the Colorado alternative system discussed earlier, where sows are not kept in stalls, the farmer argues that two months a year of confinement in farrowing crates is not onerous, given the benefit to the piglets and the sow's freedom for the remainder of the year. On the other hand, I do not believe the public will continue to accept farrowing crates in tandem with full confinement of sows during the rest of the year.

The farrowing crate raises other welfare problems besides restricted movement. Most important, perhaps, is the frustration of normal maternal behavior, an extremely powerful instinct. Sows will continue to try to make nests, even in farrowing crates. Kilgour comments: "By frustrating and stressing the sow and disallowing her maternal responses, overall productivity may not show an improvement. More research is needed."[44] Stookey echoes this sentiment: "The fact that nest building is so innate and that the sow continues to build the nest even in the absence of any material, suggests that the behavior has tremendous biological significance. No doubt survival of wild pigs is dependent upon a nest at farrowing."[45]

Thus, in my view, the primary research issue concerning farrowing crates is the development of a system that protects the piglets yet is also animal-friendly to the sow. (Indeed, the Edinburgh system displays a farrowing crate, though one with bedding.) Such a system is needed for both intensive and extensive pig rearing.[46]

Stookey recommends a system developed in Scotland by Michael Baxter and his colleagues, based on behavioral research.[47] This so-called Freedom Farrowing System allows the sow to come and go freely, but incorporates features that are attractive enough to the sow that she prefers to build her nest within the enclosure. It also includes a threshold that she can easily step over but is nearly impossible for the piglets to negotiate until they almost reach weaning. An angled false wall facilitates lying down but is designed so the piglets can escape without being crushed or trapped. In addition, a special creep area within the enclosure attracts the newborn piglets away from the center of the nest. The Freedom Farrowing System also includes a protective bar that can be lowered to lock the sow within the pad during processing of the litter. This system appears very promising and should be researched in terms of economic viability and producer acceptance.

Other alternatives have been suggested. For example, the circular crate, investigated by Frank Hurnik, could both protect the piglets and allow the sow to turn around.[48] This seems, indeed, to be an elegant solution, and further research should be given top priority.

Provision of straw or other bedding remains a problem in today's confinement systems, as mentioned earlier. Fraser argues that straw in farrowing crates would create a better situation for both mother and piglets. He also maintains that the inability of the mother to move toward the piglets in farrowing crates is frustrating for the sow, though the presence of the piglets greatly reduces confinement boredom.[49]

## Other Sow Welfare Problems

Confinement rearing of sows leads to additional welfare problems beyond those growing out of boredom, frustration, isolation, and inability to move.

Sows kept in confinement appear to have more reproductive problems, such as delay of estrus and failure of the animals to become pregnant after mating.[50] A good deal of research is needed to make these preliminary observations more precise. A 1973 study by L. Backstrom indicated that there was a higher incidence of mastitis, metritis, agalactia, prolonged farrowing time, and sow morbidity at farrowing in sows housed in confinement than in sows housed in group pens.[51] It is plausible to suggest that these negative effects are a result of prolonged stress. As Fraser points out, "In general, the coping systems of animals have evolved so as to minimize effects on reproductive success, so if there are differences between systems, even a small effect may indicate considerable welfare problems."[52]

Confined sows are more subject than unconfined sows to foot and leg problems, including the fracturing discussed briefly in Part 1. Pig farmers who have experience with both free and confined sow operations have told me that fracturing is far less common in sows that are allowed to move. Since activity is known to increase bone strength, it may well be that the immobility of confined sows renders them susceptible to leg breakage. Fraser cites work reporting a high frequency of integumental lesions in confined sows and studies going back to the 1960s showing that leg injuries, lameness, and infection are related to types of flooring.[53] Generally, slatted floors lead to more injuries than unslatted floors. Fraser remarks, "Good slats cause fewer problems than poor slats, but the incidence of sow lameness [on slats] is still very high."[54] Obviously, research into such injuries should include a search for optimum flooring.

Urinary tract disease appears to be more common in confined sows, probably because the animals lie in their excrement and because they drink less and urinate less, so that urine is more concentrated and bacteria act longer in the urinary tract. It is reasonable to attribute these problems to lack of activity, but research is needed here.

Finally, as we saw in the case of the sow with a broken leg, the combination of total confinement, automation, and the large scale of swine operations makes for minimal inspection of individual animals, sows or finishers. Thus disease and injury may be undetected until they are quite advanced, especially in sows. Further, as we saw, the minimal labor force in many operations makes treatment difficult or impossible. Unquestionably, automation tends to be inimical to stockmanship or careful husbandry. Research into modifying confinement systems to facilitate care for individual animals is necessary so that cases such as the sow with the broken leg can be handled in a humane fashion. Kilgour echoes this point when he asserts that "good stockmanship ... is especially important in large intensive units where through automation people are replaced by mechanical devices."[55]

## Piglet Welfare

A number of significant welfare problems are associated with piglets in swine production. Between day 1 and day 10 after birth, piglets are subjected to a battery of invasive procedures: vaccination, ear-notching for identification (in some cases), teeth-clipping, tail-docking, and castration of males. It is usual for producers to argue for the minimal invasiveness of these procedures, but common sense says otherwise, especially when all of them are taken together. Even if the producers are correct, public opinion is not likely to be on their side. Thus research into alternatives to these procedures is highly desirable.

Vaccination in and of itself is probably not an issue. Ear-notching, however, is surely painful, and alternatives to it exist. The microchip identification discussed earlier is probably ideal for swine, if costs can be diminished. (Visual identification of swine is not as important as it is in range cattle.) Research into dyes as a viable and inexpensive form of identification also seems reasonable.

Teeth-clipping and tail-docking are management procedures. Incisor, or "needle," teeth are clipped in order to prevent laceration of sow udders and abrasion of the faces of other piglets during competition for teats. The Universities Federation for Animal Welfare (UFAW) handbook, *Management and Welfare of Farm Animals,* argues, reasonably, that teeth-clipping should not be a routine procedure but rather should be done on an "as needed" basis, that is, where there is early evidence of damage from the teeth.[56] Given the lack of surveillance of individual animals in large intensive operations, however, the degree of scrutiny demanded by this alternative is implausible; it is simply more economical to clip routinely. Clearly, this issue should be investigated.

Docking of tails, a procedure that grew out of intensive systems, is done to prevent tail-biting, which generally increases once begun and spreads to biting other parts of the body. A victim of tail-biting gradually ceases to be reactive to being bitten, in a kind of learned helplessness. Infection often ensues and can become systemic.[57]

Pigs have always had a tendency to tail-bite. Under extensive conditions, pigs have the space to get away from one another—it is only in confinement that tail-biting became a serious problem. The response of the producer has been to amputate the distal half of the tail, a surgical solution to a humanly induced problem arising from keeping the animals in a pathogenic environment. As mentioned earlier, tail-biting is referred to as a vice, as if the pig is *bad* for tail-biting.

I do not consider surgical solutions to humanly caused animal problems morally acceptable. One ought to change the environment to a healthier one, not mutilate the animal. Fraser, following M. J. Bryant, argues that tail-biting can be prevented by changes in husbandry.[58] Animals that tend to tail-bite can be grouped together, as they do not generally show this behavior when they are so grouped. Uncomfortable atmospheric factors need to be eliminated, such as high levels of ammonia, $CO_2$, or humidity or low barometric pressure. Stocking density should be kept down. Better husbandry, provision of straw, and the opportunity to root all decrease tail-biting, according to Fraser and Broom.[59] It thus appears that boredom is relevant to tail-biting. Like other stereotypies, then, tail-biting provides a clue to conditions that need improvement. To my knowledge, no one has tried painting tails with unpleasant-tasting material to curtail biting. Such research would be cheap and easy to undertake. Even if it worked, however, the impulse leading to the behavior would remain—one would be treating symptoms.

Castration of piglets is clearly painful. As in beef cattle, castration is performed to diminish aggression and to prevent the development of adult male sexual pheromones, which give pork the "boar taint" most pork consumers dislike. Most producers agree that intact males grow better, faster, and more efficiently and produce leaner meat and more meat. It can be argued that, given the age (5–6 months) at which most males attain market weight (about 250 lb), few of the animals have reached sexual maturity. Thus the need for castration, which is expensive and painful, is obviated, especially since a pheromone test is available to detect boar-tainted carcasses. In Europe, uncastrated males are the rule. The main obstacle to eliminating castration seems to be packer resistance, based on fear of consumer rejection of boar meat and lack of packer confidence in the pheromone test. This issue is a good candidate for research that can benefit both animals and producers.

A major issue in piglet welfare arises out of early weaning. Although pigs left to their own devices will wean at 12 to 15 weeks of age, industry practice weans piglets at 3 to 4 weeks of age. As Fraser and Broom remark, "such early weaning must have considerable effects on the piglets, leading to poor welfare, but only a few have been assessed."[60] Certainly this represents a prime research issue. We know now that early weaning leads to aberrant behavior, including compulsive belly nosing and sucking, which is presumably an attempt to suck and find milk. Anal massage is a similar deviant behavior. Piglets showing this behavior chase and inflict injuries on other piglets. Other aberrant oral behavior, such as sucking on walls and bars, may also be a result of early weaning. A recent study showed that relocation of piglets to a nursery may be a major stressor augmenting early weaning. The study suggests that mixing groups of early-weaned piglets in the farrowing crate (a familiar environment) is less stressful than relocating them to a nursery.[61]

## Grower-Finishers

Increasing numbers of swine producers are operating with an "all in, all out" approach to avoid mixing of pigs, since mixing leads to stress and aggression. When pigs leave the nursery (at about 6 weeks of age), they go into a grower-finisher pen in groups of 15 to 20. One facility I visited placed them in a pen 8 feet by 25 feet. They remain together for the next five or so months until reaching market weight. Groups of fifteen to twenty allow the pigs to establish a stable hierarchy. At the early stages of finishing, the pen seems to provide adequate space, but by the time the pigs attain market weight, they appear to be quite crowded. Given the ethic we have discussed, I believe the public would consider the pigs too crowded. Research should be undertaken to determine the cost of providing additional space.

Austere environments in grower-finisher pens represent another welfare problem that may augment tail-biting. It is true, as producers argue, that the pigs have one another to interact with as a check against boredom, and they do play a great deal. Typically, though, the animals are not given toys (such as bowling balls) as an additional deterrent to boredom, because such devices can damage pens. This lack may well lead to boredom-based tail-biting and aggression. Research should be undertaken into enriching the environment in ways that do not work against the system. Provision of straw would be a step toward an enriched environment. Access to the outdoors and to dirt, as discussed with regard to sows, might also represent an enriched environment for finishers kept indoors.

As mentioned earlier, access to the outdoors raises feed costs. On the other hand, such access might counter some of the untoward effects of indoor finishing, such as high humidity, poor ventilation, and problems with respiratory disease. According to Fox, "it has been found that 35 to 60 percent of all pigs raised in confinement buildings are affected with mycoplasmic pneumonia to the point where weight gain is adversely affected."[62] In numerous pig facilities, workers must wear respirators; obviously, such a situation is harmful to human and animal welfare. Modified open-front buildings, which may be a workable alternative to total confinement,[63] should be studied in terms of economic viability.

Another problem appears to be lighting, which is both short in duration and low in intensity. Pigs are kept in limited lighting to avoid aggression yet will work to obtain light. Research into optimal lighting should be undertaken and systems devised to meet those needs. Light cycles have major physiological consequences.

Amount of space per pig is important. Equally important is *quality* of space. Space in grower-finisher pens should take account of the need or desire of pigs for separate dunging and lying facilities, for eating without harassment by others, and for ways of avoiding attack. As we saw, meeting these concerns is a major component of the Edinburgh-Stolba system. The provision of "hidey-holes" for pigs has been shown to reduce untoward effects of aggression.[64]

Foot and leg problems associated with problematic flooring are another area of concern. Slippery floors can cause lameness, abrasions, strains, and foot injuries. Slats may lead to trapped and broken claws. Some preference work on flooring has been done, but as Fraser points out, it should be followed by studies of welfare and injury on the various types of floors.[65] Much research has been carried out on flooring, but a definitive synthesis has yet to be made.

## Handling and Transport

Being highly intelligent and sensitive animals, pigs are very responsive to stressors.[66] Handling is thus relevant to productivity. Indeed, in two separate studies, Paul Hemsworth and H. W. Gonyou have shown that pigs receiving positive handling and interaction are easier to manage, have faster growth rates, and have better reproductive success than pigs receiving negative handling.[67]

In research and on farms, those handling pigs often rely on "macho muscling" methods, which produce significant stress. It is far better, as the National Pork Producers Council *Swine Care Handbook* states, to employ knowledge of pig behavior for handling.[68] Hotshot use should be minimal—most pigs can be handled and moved without it by "pig smart" people. The establishment of seminars in handling of the sort done by Temple Grandin would benefit both animals and producers.

Transportation is a major stressor for an animal kept in confinement all its life and suddenly moved outside, loaded, and transported. Grandin has shown that pigs raised in environments that have some stimulation (suspended plastic tubing) move and load easier than those raised in barren environments, presumably because they have learned to deal with some variety.[69]

Grandin points out that restriction of sensory input makes the nervous system more reactive to stimulation. This is important, because loading has been shown to be a greater stressor than transport. Mixing of pigs during transport is also a significant stressor, as is poor, rough driving.

Ignoring the stresses of loading, handling, and transport can lead to bruising, carcass blemishes, PSE (Pale Soft Exudative) syndrome, and malignant hyperthermia syndrome, all of which harm both producers and animals. Research into "idiot-proof" systems of loading, handling, and transport would therefore be of great value.

## Other Issues

Continued, sophisticated research into swine behavior and cognition should be supported.[70] I believe that the better we understand the "mind of the pig," the more we will be able to grasp the subtleties of making production systems animal-friendly. Good research may be expensive, but we need a research scalpel, as it were, not a bludgeon. The sort of work done by Stolba and Wood-Gush could be refined considerably. It would be reasonable for USDA to hire a full-time swine behaviorist to work on understanding the animal well enough to put that knowledge to practical use.

A final welfare problem that has not yet been recognized by the industry is the increasing prevalence of hyperexcitable pigs, described by Grandin.[71] The animals squeal when touched, show an extreme flocking instinct, and are difficult to move or handle even by experts. The animals are costly to the industry because they show high levels of PSE. Pigs selected for leanness and muscling seem to have the greatest tendency toward hyperexcitability, which is exacerbated by lack of environmental stimulation. Research into the genetic and environmental basis of this problem should be a top priority.

# 5 The Dairy Industry

Historically, probably no area of traditional, extensive, preindustrial agriculture realized the contractual, "we take care of the animals, the animals take care of us" ethic more than dairy farming. What made dairy an especially good example of the contract between animal and human was the early realization that gentle, compassionate treatment of cattle leads to significantly better milk yield. Science has recently confirmed what common sense already knew—that the variable correlating most highly with milk production is the personality of the herder and that women generally make the best stock managers.[1]

Thus, while few people considered range beef cattle members of the family, as it were, such was not the case with dairy cows. A colleague of mine who grew up on an extensive dairy farm recalls that there was no bigger honor in his family than to be named after one of the favored cows. Students still tell me that their fathers cried after the death of a favorite cow. Since dairy cattle were raised for their products, not their meat, the element of killing was not central to such farming, and animals often lived for a long time, even beyond what could be justified by productivity alone.

This view of dairy entered popular culture and, in my view, still makes the general public favorably disposed toward milk production. The image of "Bessy" happily chewing her cud is a cliché, often depicted in cartoons, and the Carnation Company has indelibly stamped an entire generation or two with the pastoral picture of "contented cows." Few members of the general public would agree with the activist statement I heard at an animal welfare conference: "I can think of nothing more disgusting than drinking the milk of another species." The dairy industry would be wise to confirm this perception of concern, not erode it.[2]

One of the most dramatic changes in dairies, directly relevant to public perception of the industry, is the rise of large, intensive dairy operations, with up to three thousand cattle maintained in relatively small acreages. The small dairy farmer, with names for his cows, is a vanishing breed, as land costs, labor costs, and capital investment costs increase. The public tends, with some justification, to equate large operations with lack of concern and attention to individual animals. On the other hand, proponents of large, well-capitalized, intensive operations argue that their dairies, unlike small ones, are able to afford sufficient labor to look after the cows and actually provide for more inspection of the animals, since mechanization and automation have removed much of the "scut" work. C. W. Arave and J. L. Albright have argued that this is true for mastitis control.[3] Supporting this view is the fact that, unlike sows, cows are relatively expensive and highly productive (the modern cow can produce 10,000 to 36,000 pounds of milk per year),[4] and thus careful attention to the animal also benefits the producer. Albright has maintained that mechanization is no substitute for stockmanship, a point echoed by others.[5] Research into this question would be highly desirable; if it is true that large dairies do pay attention to individual animals, such research could blunt negative public perceptions of these operations. If it is false, the research would probably lead to revisions in industry practice and to better management. Such investigations might compare small and large dairies in terms of various parameters related to welfare. My key point is that, regardless of size of operation, concern for individual animals is still operative.

One area which feeds the idea of callousness at large dairies is the treatment of surplus calves. My colleague, Temple Grandin, informs me that such calves often receive no colostrum, and are shipped as young as one day old, before they can even ambulate properly.

In this chapter, we discuss a variety of researchable welfare issues in the dairy industry, some of which are real and some of which may be a function of untutored perceptions. In either case, however, these problems must be laid to rest. As those in the animal industry often remark, in animal welfare, perception is reality. Unfortunately, as Albright has forcefully pointed out, "very little organized U.S. research on dairy animal welfare is under way. A library CRIS-USDA computer search from 1978–1986 with such key words as dairy, cattle, cow, calves, calf, veal, welfare, humane, or well-being revealed four projects active and pertinent to this discussion."[6]

Although the raising of so-called white veal is a spinoff of the dairy industry, this subject is discussed in the next chapter.

## Ethograms for Cattle

There is an urgent need for fundamental research into the

normal behavior patterns of modern dairy cattle under the open conditions for which they were historically selected, something like what was achieved at Edinburgh for domestic swine. Unfortunately, there is no wild population of *Bos taurus* analogous to the population of European wild swine that Stolba used as a basis for ethological comparisons. The closest analogue may be beef cattle maintained under range conditions or dairy cattle still kept under traditional conditions. At any rate, methodology must be devised and research conducted that will provide researchers with a baseline "ethogram" of natural behavior for dairy cattle, which can then be used to assess current systems. Such research would be invaluable for welfare concerns. In addition, as Temple Grandin and others have shown, knowledge of fundamental behavior is useful for handling and management. As we noted earlier, behavior seems to be emerging as a focal point for welfare deliberations. At the same time, cattle exhibit fewer stereotypies than other animals but do show some. It has been suggested that cud-chewing provides a built-in form of self-stimulation that allows the animal to cope with austere environments, even as gum-chewing has carried generations of students through boring lectures.

## Calf Welfare

Some of the major potential hot spots for the industry come from the treatment of calves. Most female calves are used as replacements for dairy cows. Various practices associated with raising such calves have been criticized on welfare grounds.

One such issue is the early separation of calf from mother. Common sense suggests that such a separation is stressful to both animals, since cattle under extensive conditions can suckle for some seven months. According to Albright, such separation is necessary in order to expedite human-cow interaction; cattle reared by dams or by nurse cows with no human involvement "are more difficult to calm down, have greater flight distances, ... circle continuously in the holding pen, and are difficult to train to the milking routine."[7] In other words, the early stress of separation may improve the welfare of the animal later when it becomes a dairy cow, since humans have become "surrogate mothers" to the calves, as Albright puts it.[8] On the other hand, the average person sees removing a baby from its mother as paradigmatically abusive, even cruel.

It is obvious that the practice of separating calves at an early age from mothers should be further researched, with regard to stress on both cow and calf and ways of mitigating that stress. Since virtually all dairy farmers effect such separation, the issue has considerable significance.

A related question concerns the optimal time for removing calf from cow. This is currently disputed, most notably with respect to the provision of colostrum. Some dairy farmers leave the calf with the mother for up to three days to allow the calf to suckle, to permit a mother-offspring relationship to form, and to render the cow's milk free of colostrum and thus able to be sold. In contrast, others separate the calf immediately and deliver the colostrum through a nipple-pail or bottle.

Although it may seem more humane to allow the cow and calf the longer period to bond, one can argue that separation of the calf after three days, rather than at birth, causes greater trauma. According to Albright:

> When the calf is left with the cow three days or more, it is more difficult to separate the pair. Excessive bawling, fussing, and breaking down fences occur when maternal urges are then denied, and the cow will fret excessively when separated from the calf, resulting in decreased milk production.[9]

This observation points again toward the need for further research in minimizing the stress of separation. It is also clear that close attention to separation of calf from dam by the public could generate bad publicity for the industry, given the sanctity of the mother-offspring relationship for common sense. Research into raising calves on nurse cows, as is sometimes done in the beef industry, should perhaps be undertaken. Dairy bulls raised on nurse cows grow up less dangerous, because they never lose their fear of humans.

Another welfare issue concerns the housing of calves. In the United States, it is most common to raise calves for about three months in individual pens or hutches to which the calf may be tethered. Although such hutches are an improvement over crates, since animals in fenced-in hutches can move freely, they are still offensive to many people, who dislike the restricted space and isolation from other animals. Despite the fact that probably the primary purpose of individual housing is disease prevention and ease of observing individuals, many dairymen allow calves to interact with others in adjacent pens or hutches. J. H. B. Roy has argued that calves are happier when they can see one another,[10] and most dairymen with whom I have discussed this issue agree. Outside hutches reduce calf mortality over inside ones.

Supporters of individual housing argue that dairy calves "do better and develop normally if they are kept individually until weaning,"[11] especially in outdoor pens. They cite higher survival rates, less disease, and reduced tendency for persistent intersucking among calves raised this way. Albright has maintained that the "vice" of intersucking, which is prevalent in Europe, is a function of early group housing.[12]

A different view is expressed by Ronald Kilgour and Clive Dalton, who favorably cite work by H. H. Sambraus to justify "the importance of keeping calves in groups to ensure appropriate resting behavior, social and activity behavior ... the calf's surroundings should provide plenty of stimuli to allow exploration and play."[13]

Similarly, Fraser asserts that "individually reared calves cannot interact much with one another and long periods of social isolation lead to failure to develop normal social behavior."[14]

Strangely enough, some research has shown that calves raised in isolation, though indeed subject to a chronic stressor, nevertheless produce more milk as adults.[15] This conclusion is open to many interpretations, ranging from the simple notion that individual productivity is not a mark of welfare, to the complex idea suggested by Albright that "isolation stress has an organizational effect on the ontogeny of the hypothalamo-hypophysial-adrenal system of neonatal calves. The resultant stronger response to adult stressors could increase milk production."[16]

In general, given diversity of opinion as well as the strong tendency of the nonagricultural public to react negatively to isolation of calves, research should continue in this area. Ideally, group systems should be developed that do everything isolation does but allow the calves to enjoy social interaction. According to Fraser, "with further refinement of management procedures, ... [straw-based] systems are likely to [become] ... the normal method of calf housing."[17] We discuss calf welfare further in Chapter 6, which deals with the veal industry.

## Welfare Issues of Cows

### Housing Systems

The dairy industry in the United States employs a wide variety of housing systems for dairy cattle, ranging from highly extensive, very traditional pasture systems to stanchion or tie-stall housing to free-stall housing. Positive and negative features relevant to welfare are associated with all systems, but some seem more problematic than others. The system of greatest concern is probably tie stalls, where the animals are tied in one place for long periods of time. Tie stalls are used almost exclusively in the Midwest and Northeast. Although the apparent historical motivation for tie stalls was concern for the well-being of the cattle as well as reduction of labor, with tie stalls allowing for ease of observation and inspection of the cows,[18] the fact that the animals are unable to move and unable to engage in normal behavior, notably grooming, makes tie stalls a plausible and inevitable target for social concern. Whereas a range cow walks more than 6,000 meters a day,[19] a cow in a tie stall is clearly prevented from such exercise. In addition, the cow's social nature is frustrated by such housing systems. Getting up and lying down can also be a problem in poorly designed stalls. Many tie-stall operators let the cows out onto pasture or dry lots for one to five hours a day when weather permits but keep them inside during bad weather.

Many dairy cattle, especially in the West, are kept in dry-lot conditions, in outdoor dirt pens in groups. The cow can express her social nature and can exercise. The problems with dry lots are similar to problems with feedlots: lack of shade, lack of shelter from wind and snow, poor drainage, and general lack of protection from climatic extremes. Some farmers do provide shade and cooling with sprinklers. In general, cattle withstand cold stress better than heat stress.

Free stalls have gained in popularity since their invention in 1960. In such systems, the cows can be in their own bedded stalls and move freely into concrete or earth yards where they receive food and water. Poor flooring in these systems can lead to foot and leg problems. Given a choice, dairy cattle prefer other flooring over concrete.[20] Research is needed into flooring that reduces slippage and injury and into more effective sanitizing systems for waste removal. Poor hygiene in the stalls can also cause mastitis and is an issue that should be addressed.

One problem with all these systems is that they fail to allow for grazing on pasture, an activity for which cattle have evolved and which, if permitted, they will spend eight to ten hours a day doing.[21] (Indeed, one can argue that the domestication of cattle resulted precisely from their ability to convert forage into food consumable by humans.) Swedish legislation aimed at respecting the rights of animals following from their biological natures has stressed the need for cattle to graze and indeed granted cattle the right to graze in perpetuity.[22] It is likely that public opinion in the United States similarly favors the grazing of cattle; few pastoral images are as powerful and pervasive as that of cows on pasture.

Some farmers pasture dry cows, but the keeping of milking cows on pasture has diminished, except in areas of the Southeast where climate and rainfall favor lush growth. Arave and Albright have pointed out that pasturing raises its own problems.[23] In northern states, the grazing season is limited. Pasture may not supply the consistent quality and quantity of nutrients required by high-producing cows. Other problems cited by Arave and Albright include shade, heat, water, insects, bloat, and energy wasted in movement. Although many farmers believe that cattle prefer pasture to other feedstuffs, Kilgour cites research showing that pasture ranked ninth of twenty in a preference study.[24] Albright has proposed research into the feasibility of incorporating pasturing into modern dairy systems, which seems indeed to be a major welfare and economic research priority.[25]

In general, research into housing and management systems that respect the cow's physical and behavioral nature, while encouraging productivity and health, needs to be carried out for the dairy industry. The elimination of total confinement systems such as tie stalls should take precedence in this category.

## Castration, Dehorning, and Branding

As in beef cattle, dehorning is a problem, as is castration of bull calves; both issues have already been discussed. Most operators do not brand dairy cattle.

## Tail-docking

Docking of tails in dairy cows has gained in popularity in the United States and Canada. It is alleged that tail-docking reduces mastitis and somatic cell counts (SCC). The docking is often accomplished by elastrators, described in the discussion of beef cattle castration. Allegedly, the procedure is painless and keeps the cow from flinging manure.

Conversations with dairy specialists, dairy veterinarians, and a lactation physiologist have convinced me that there is absolutely no scientific basis for claims about the benefits of tail-docking. Problems with mastitis are largely a function of hygiene, arising when animals are regularly down in unclean stalls. Removing the tail is another example of attempting to handle a problem of human management by mutilating the animal—as in "devocalization" of dogs, declawing of cats, and docking tails in piglets. In this situation, however, unlike the others, the procedure does not even solve the problem. Indeed, removing the tail causes suffering to the cow, since it can no longer deal with flies!

Not only is docking the tail, in fact, not curative; it can exacerbate the problem. The use of elastrators, contrary to the belief of some farmers, is quite painful. The procedure can also cause infection, death, and decreased milk production. In purely prudential risk-benefit terms, then, it is irrational to choose to dock the tails, and since there is no potential benefit from the procedure, the farmer is not rationally warranted in taking any risk whatsoever. The same point, of course, holds for surgical docking of the tail.

Indeed, there is reason to believe that docking the tails is likely to increase the very problem that the farmer is trying to eliminate, namely, high somatic cell counts. Kilgour and others have reported that stress elevates SCC in dairy cattle,[26] and the use of the elastrator and the subsequent pain and distress that it causes the animal certainly represent a stressor, as does any ensuing infection. Furthermore, since stress results in immunosuppression, an animal experiencing the docking procedure is surely more prone than ever to mastitis, since its immune system is being compromised.

It appears to me that the noninvasive alternative of clipping the tail switch should work as well as docking, if there is anything to the theory implicating tails in mastitis. The issue should definitely be researched as a welfare concern.

## Mastitis and Lameness

According to Fraser and Broom, lameness and mastitis are the two major welfare problems in dairy cattle and there is a positive correlation between the incidence of these diseases.[27] Lameness has in turn been tied to high-protein and high-concentrate diets.[28] Lameness can be reduced by hoof trimming and foot baths and by attention to flooring,[29] but "much remains to be discovered about the conditions which lead to individuals being likely to become lame."[30] A good deal of lameness is a result of laminitis. This collection of issues should be studied in tandem with research into improving stall housing and controlling mastitis.[31] Many of these problems can currently be handled with good husbandry and "cow smart" labor—the challenge, as in all modern agriculture, is to make the systems "idiot-proof." Research into better flooring, waste disposal, sanitation, and diet would help create systems that are animal-friendly even when stockmanship is not perfect.

## Downer Animals

The dairy industry is probably the primary source of "downer" animals, discussed earlier in this book. While increasing numbers of dairymen are beginning to realize that nothing is more erosive to the "contented cow" image of the dairy industry than transporting and then dragging a downer cow with a tractor or loader to the kill floor, other elements of the industry have turned a blind eye to the problem. Most dairy downers are probably a result of calcium-phosphorus imbalance leading to milk fever (hypocalcemia). Animals that are down should be killed on the farm and not transported. The industry should deal with this issue before it is legislated—both state and federal initiatives are pending regarding downer animals.

## The Human Environment

Much knowledge has accumulated, based on both practical experience and science, regarding human interaction with dairy cattle. This variable is fundamental both to milk production and to cow well-being. Cattle are creatures of habit, and disruption of habits can be highly stressful. Indeed, Kilgour has shown that introduction into a new environment is more stressful for cattle than electric shock.[32] Good stockmen respect this aspect of cow handling. One successful dairy farmer has asserted:

Handling the dairy cow requires patience and skill, neither of which is learned overnight. Milkers must work at a pace to which the cows are accustomed. After a routine has been set, the cow will usually accept it. This means no drastic changes can be made over a short period of time. Even changing the ration must be done slowly to allow the cow time to adjust.[33]

M. F. Seabrook has shown that the personality of the herder is the most significant variable in high milk production.[34] A good livestock manager can detect deviations from habitual behavior that indicate environmental, feeding, or disease problems. Seabrook has detailed the variety of ways in which interactions with humans influence cattle and pigs, an area that is a fertile field for further research.[35] Albright has summarized some of the relevant features of a good herdsman (or woman; there is some evidence that women, often being gentler, are better cow caretakers).[36] Obviously, research aimed at articulating the best elements of stockmanship is desirable.

Additional research into cow handling and facilities design based on knowledge of cow behavior is also warranted. Temple Grandin, a pioneer in this area, has done much to develop animal-friendly handling systems, yet her results are typically underused.[37] For example, she has shown that solid-sided chutes work better than open-sided ones, that uniform illumination (rather than patterns of light, shadow, and darkness) prevents balking, and that floor surface affects ease of movement, yet many farmers have not incorporated these insights into their facilities.

## Future Technology

New technology is moving quickly into the dairy industry. Technological innovation can have significant implications for the well-being of the animals. Consequently, all new technology must be evaluated in terms of welfare at the same time as it is being developed for productivity and efficiency.

The rise of automated computerized milking should be carefully monitored. It has been argued that this technology

could allow the elimination of the milking parlor, because cows could at their leisure enter stalls to be milked automatically. More frequent milking would increase production and place less stress on the udder. An important benefit would be to allow the stockman to spend more time observing and tending his animals and less time on routine laborious work.[38]

On the other hand, such an innovation could go wrong in many ways, lead to less attention to the animals, and further erode the bond between humans and farm animals.

Genetic engineering can also cause problems. Recent work on double muscling led to unexplained weakness and paralysis in the calves.[39] Other animals (pigs and chickens) engineered for increased size have shown a variety of problems, notably with feet and legs, since foot and leg strength did not increase in proportion to the additional size. Cloned calves have been extremely large at birth, leading to birthing difficulties, and have shown other problems, including alleged "stupidity."[40] As discussed earlier, in all genetic engineering programs the resultant animals should be no worse off than their parent stock and should be carefully monitored.

The use of BST (discussed in Chapter 2) and similar growth hormone innovations developed through biotechnology should also be evaluated for effect on cattle well-being. It has been argued that the use of BST will amplify a problem already prevalent in the dairy industry as a result of artificial insemination.[41] In evaluating AI sires (bulls whose semen is used for artificial insemination), a major criterion is the first lactation production of the bulls' daughters:

> Unfortunately, a bull may be bred to thousands of cows before an evaluation can be made of the longevity of his daughters. The result is strong selection pressure for high first lactation production and weak selection pressure for longevity, a major factor in efficient production. We are thus selecting for a 100 metre dash cow, forgetting that the most profitable cow is the marathon cow.[42]

Thus many cows are culled during the third lactation, before they reach their (theoretically highest) fifth lactation. BST could augment this problem. Canadian research showed that "BST treatment was associated with an increased culling rate presumably as a result of increased stress associated with higher milk production."[43] The study showed that while BST increased milk production by 14.4 percent, it increased the culling rate by 45 percent. According to this argument,

> This dramatic rise in the culling rate as a result of the injection of BST is further confirmation that we have through natural selection, bred cows to produce a level of BST which jeopardizes their chances of surviving until their most productive years. Injecting additional BST makes matters worse.[44]

The use of BST also makes the cows more prone to mastitis,[45] perhaps because the animals are giving more milk and the lactation ducts are more patent and thus more susceptible to bacterial invasion.[46]

The dairy industry, by and large, has not been the target of negative publicity, except as the source of downer cattle. The problems we have discussed should be aggressively researched in order to preserve the industry's enviable position in the public mind.

# 6 The Veal Industry

White veal production is to animal agriculture as the Draize test (where cosmetics or shampoos are put into rabbits' eyes to test for irritancy) is to animal research. Both are perceived by the public as examples of these activities at their worst. Like placing potential irritants into rabbits' eyes and scoring the resultant lesions for the sake of generating new cosmetics, what is seen as "torturing" calves to produce an expensive product consumed by a small portion of the population is unacceptable to the social ethic. I would guess that the average person sees white veal as a decadent product, analogous to the pâté de foie gras produced by force-feeding geese whose feet have been nailed to a board. Insofar as white veal is a symbol to the public at large of the worst in industrialized agriculture, it seems reasonable—indeed, critical—for agriculture to address veal production promptly and forthrightly, and to modify it so that it is consonant with the new ethic for animals.

My own experiences with public attitudes toward veal provide, I believe, a typical reflection of opinion. I travel and lecture extensively and mingle with a wide cross-section of the population, from ranchers to urbanites, from blue-collar workers to college presidents. It is noteworthy that, across these populations, it is ethically correct—and mainstream—to assert that one does not eat veal, on humane grounds. Refusing to eat veal is not fringe or flaky; it is acceptable, exactly on a par with refusing to wear fur. John Gibbons, the president's science advisor, recently declared publicly that he does not eat veal for ethical reasons.[1] A high USDA official told me that he, and about half his peers, similarly will not eat veal. The vast majority of western ranchers I talk to also disavow veal on ethical grounds.

Some years ago, I had a striking experience that underscores this point. I had been asked by the Colorado commissioner of agriculture to participate in a seminar on the issues of animal rights and animal welfare for the leaders of Colorado agriculture. Among the speakers was a drug company executive representing the Animal Industry Foundation, a group devoted to opposing the animal rights movement. He began his presentation by showing a short video called "The Other Side of the Fence," produced by the ASPCA. The video is highly critical of white veal production, arguing that just as human babies have needs, so do calves. Though we try to meet the needs of babies, we do not in the case of calves used for veal. His stated purpose in showing the tape was to demonstrate the sophisticated level of propaganda directed by animal groups against animal agriculture, in order to galvanize the audience into opposing such activity. A few hours later, I sat at lunch with the head of the Colorado Farm Bureau and the president of the Colorado Cattlemen's Association. I asked them for their reaction to the film. The Cattlemen's Association president replied as follows: "Well, it brought tears to my eyes. There is no cause to raise animals that way. If people want veal, we can kill some calves. We don't have to torture them. If I had to raise animals that way, I'd get the hell out of the business." The others at the table concurred.

This was not an isolated incident. I have yet to address a group of cattle ranchers who find the production of white veal acceptable. Indeed, if I were to transcribe the remarks generally made by the ranchers about veal into a typescript, one would probably assume from the text that one was reading the opinions of extreme animal rightists! (I actually have such a transcript, based on a seminar I gave in Worland, Wyoming.)

One could argue that the strong antipathy toward white veal production in the general public is a function of emotionalism, sentimentality, the "Bambi syndrome," the fact that calves have "big soulful eyes," and the like. But such a claim can surely not be made about ranchers. In their case, the distaste for veal production is a result of their understanding of the cattle telos, and their belief that nothing could be further from accommodating that telos than the raising of white veal.

Finally, one finds similar repugnance among leading scientists whose fields are farm animal welfare and ethology. Andrew Fraser, arguably the world's best farm animal ethologist, and author of the classic *Farm Animal Behaviour and Welfare,* has asserted: "Since white veal production is inefficient and there are inevitable welfare problems, it is to be hoped that public demand for it will continue its rapid downward trend and such production systems will soon disappear."[2] John Webster, author of *Calf Husbandry, Health, and Welfare*[3] and probably the leading British authority on calf welfare, has condemned the raising of white veal as follows:

> Man has a responsibility to rear the farm animals that give him his living in an ethically acceptable manner. The rearing of a calf for veal in a confined crate with a slatted floor on a diet of milk replacer alone has been considered

ethically unacceptable by many people of reasonable opinion. One should not expect such people to produce an argument as long and as detailed as this booklet to support their views. If, in a democratic society, a majority of people decide that a particular practice is unacceptable and their politicians agree, then unacceptable it is. The scientist can no more determine what is and is not acceptable than any other individual. He can only offer glimpses of the truth in the hope that they will influence the ethical decisions of reasonable people. Such glimpses of the truth as are offered in this booklet lend strong support to popular criticisms of veal production, since we have demonstrated that to confine calves in individual boxes on slatted floors and feed them entirely on a liquid diet abnormally low in iron abuses each of the "five freedoms."

It is, therefore, imperative that more acceptable methods of rearing calves for veal be developed.[4]

Note that none of the people cited above are at all opposed to the raising of animals for meat or even to raising calves for meat. They are opposed rather to the current *manner* of raising veal. They all believe that veal can be raised in a morally acceptable way. As we shall see, Webster has described a system for doing so.

## Welfare Problems in Current Systems

### Behavioral Deprivation

In an exhaustive paper published in *Applied Animal Behavior Science* in 1988, T. H. Friend and G. R. Dellmeier discuss the behavioral deprivation associated with current systems of veal production.[5] They point out that "research has identified positive correlation between the degree of behavioral deprivation and physiological responses indicative of chronic stress, increased disease incidence and behavioral anomalies."[6] In their discussion of housing systems, they take as their point of departure the ethogram for cattle, that is,

Table 6.1.  **Major bovine ethogram components affected by calf housing and management systems**

| | |
|---|---|
| General postural behavior | Social behavior |
| Ingestive behavior | Explorative behavior |
| Locomotion/kinesis | Reproductive behavior |
| Sleeping/resting | Eliminative behavior |
| Body maintenance/grooming | Circadian/diurnal rhythms |

*Source:* T. H. Friend and G. R. Dellmeier, "Common Practices and Problems Related to Artificially Rearing Calves: An Ethological Analysis," *Applied Animal Behavior Science* 20(1988):48. Reprinted with permission.

the comprehensive behavioral catalog for the species (Table 6.1).

By appealing to this table, one can assess the limitations of various systems. Friend and Dellmeier point out that "veal crates are an extreme example of maximum close individual confinement with significant curtailment of a variety of natural behaviors. Most of the behaviors listed on Table 6.1 are restricted, if not totally prevented, by this method."[7] For example, such calves exhibit increased motivation for locomotion and social behavior and have a greater incidence of impaired locomotor ability.[8] Fraser and Broom point out that the calves are housed in small enclosures where they cannot turn around and cannot groom the hind portion of their bodies, which calves normally do several times a day. This leads to significant frustration. Consequently, the calves groom excessively those parts of the body that they can reach, which in turn results in hairballs in the rumen.[9]

Lying behavior is important for cattle. In crates, calves cannot assume certain standardly adopted lying postures, another deprivation that serves as a source of frustration.[10] Not surprisingly, then, calves show a good deal of stereotypical behavior, a sign, as we discussed, of poor welfare.[11] As Friend points out, these behavioral indicators are buttressed by measures of both long- and short-term physiological stress responses.[12]

Friend also stresses the thwarting of social behavior and play. He reminds us that social interaction is known to be a source of both physical and physiological comfort and that play, which in calves is largely social, is a "sensitive indicator of overall general psychological as well as physical well-being."[13] A similar point is true of exploration.

Friend argues a point applicable to all confinement agriculture, an observation also made by M. W. Fox.[14] A sense of control—or even prediction—is essential to all animals, as we noted in the discussion of Hal Markowitz's approach to behavioral enrichment. Confinement robs animals of control, which in turn diminishes their ability to cope with stressors.[15] A confined animal has no control and cannot cope; it cannot scratch an itch, stretch a leg, chase a fly, or run from a perceived threat. This situation could result in a form of learned helplessness, a morally unacceptable state in animals extensively studied by M. E. P. Seligman and others as a model for human depression.[16] If we are in effect creating learned helplessness in veal calves, this is a prima facie reason to condemn such a system.

## Diet

Two major dietary welfare problems are associated with the raising of white veal. First, because veal calves are "milk fed," that is, fed only milk or milk replacer and no roughage, the rumen and its microflora develop unnaturally, often resulting in abomasal ulcers and predisposing the animal to enteritis and indigestion from hairballs.[17] On the other hand, Webster reports that calves fed dry rations and calves kept on straw had nearly 100 percent incidence of abomasal ulcers. Webster feels that these ulcers cause no harm.[18] Obviously, further research is needed to resolve these conflicting views. According to Fraser and Broom, calves should be fed adequate roughage from the second week of life, a diet that would also help eliminate some behavioral anomalies growing out of the animals' failure to achieve oral satisfaction.[19]

Second, in order to obtain white veal, producers must strictly limit the iron intake of the calves. The redness of beef is a function of haem compounds, which contain iron. Myoglobin is the haem compound in muscle; hemoglobin is the compound in blood. Webster has pointed out that one cannot produce white veal without feeding a diet that will certainly produce anemia in some calves.[20] This is the case whether the calves are raised in crates or in groups; indeed, Webster has argued that the meat from calves kept in groups with straw tended to be whiter than that of calves in boxes, perhaps because ingestion of straw interfered with iron absorption.[21]

An additional dietary problem generated by confinement rearing grows out of the system of feeding. Usually, the animals are fed twice a day from a bucket. This frustrates their normal sucking behavior and leads to behavioral anomalies. Furthermore, the animals tend to consume much more milk at the two feedings than they would consume at any of the four to ten feedings they would have if nursing, which in turn can cause digestive problems.

## Flooring

Slatted floors are uncomfortable and severely restrict behavior.

## Group Housing

It would appear prima facie that group housing of veal calves on straw would be the solution to many of the problems enumerated above. However, group, or loose, housing presents its own problems. In particular, group-raised calves tend to show intersucking and urine drinking.[22] Also, less aggressive calves may not receive proper amounts of feed. Such problems may be resolved by use of a computer-controlled, transponder-activated system, developed by Webster, which allows individual calves to eat controlled amounts several times a day.[23]

A 1992 study by D. D. Johnson and colleagues reported on a group housing system and demonstrated that meat color, type of management system (i.e., group housing versus pen), and diet (milk versus grain) had no effect on palatability.[24] If anything, research has shown that as pigment increased, flavor became more intense.[25] H. A. Agboola and others have argued that provision of monosodium phosphate and vitamin E late in veal feeding can be used to "regulate tissue Fe and myoglobin synthesis and to produce lighter colored veal without making the calf anemic."[26] Electrical stimulation of carcasses also improves lean color.[27]

The disadvantages of group housing systems as perceived by the industry are summarized in a 1987 article by T. J. Seubert published in the *Vealer*:

> There is greater disease transmission due to calf interaction, sleeping on the same bedding, and drinking from the same source. Death losses are "as much as doubled," and there is a 25 percent greater incidence of health problems. It is more difficult to observe calves and their feces individually. Respiratory disease conditions are increased by bedding and higher ammonia. Calves do not finish out uniformly. Greater excitement occurs when an animal must be removed or treated.[28]

## Research Issues

The research priorities in the veal industry are patent. First and foremost, research should be aimed at refining our extant knowledge of group housing so as to avoid the current problems, make it cost-effective, and respond to the vealers' concerns described above, notably disease problems.

Such research should aim at systems that allow the animals to express their natural behaviors. Feeding systems should have proper nutrition and schedules that avoid the causing of behavioral aberrations. A major priority for research is pursuing methods of preserving white meat while not rendering the animal anemic, by either dietary means (as in the use of phosphates and vitamin E) or carcass treatment. Alternatively, research aimed at educating the public about the irrelevance of white as opposed to pink or red veal to palatability and tenderness could be undertaken, although this strategy is less likely to be effective.

Crated, anemic, or borderline-anemic veal is no longer acceptable to the social ethic. If the veal industry is to survive, it must change dramatically.

Trevor Tomkins, vice-president of Quantock, the British company that pioneered loose housing in the 1970s, has discussed the need for the sort of reforms we have noted. He indicates that the industry started off on the wrong foot in the 1950s, with systems quickly developed to deal with a surplus of calves and skim milk.

> It was only natural that attempts should be made to feed that skim milk back to calves. Knowledge of the nutrient requirements of the calf were poor, and the calves were fed far from a balanced diet. The consequence was poor performance, high disease levels, and high mortality. The only way to control

the problem was to isolate calves in individual crates to prevent severe cross-infection and to make treatment easier. The consequence was that the veal industry started to develop with "the cart before the horse" from the outset. But it is only with hindsight coupled with thirty years of research into the nutrition and husbandry of the young calf that we are aware of that mistake. *Clearly it is unnatural for any young animal to be raised in isolation,* but now modern practice allows real and economically viable alternatives.

All of us in this industry are aware that the animal rights issue is one which has in the past and will in the future become an area of major debate. None of us should lose sight of the power that such debate has to influence the economics and viability of our industry. ... The pressure from animal rights groups will continue to grow until ultimately there is a balance between what people see as acceptable methods of raising animals and what is dictated by sound objective science in terms of animal health and profit for the veal producer. Loose housing managed properly and set up with professional advice based on real experience does offer profit to the producers and will at the same time help quiet those critics of the veal industry who are concerned about the way animals are raised and treated. The quote from Professor John Webster, who is one of the leading influences in modern production research in Europe, sums it up. "It is, I think, reasonable to assume that man and cattle will continue their relationship as long as both species survive. It is equally reasonable to conclude that, as man determines the nature of this relationship, he has an obligation to ensure reasonable standards of welfare for the animals in his charge, which means a reasonable life according to (1) hunger and malnutrition, (2) thermal and physical discomfort, (3) injury and disease, (4) suppression of 'normal' behavior, (5) fear and stress."[29]

By forthrightly meeting social concerns about animal welfare, the veal industry could turn what is an appalling weakness into a strength and make its product much more socially acceptable. As Tomkins puts it, "with a little more sharing of ideas and less dependence on fiction, the American veal industry could become the shining example to the livestock sector of the agricultural industry, and loose housing will be seen as a profitable alternative in what is currently an industry with problems."[30] Failure to act could, on the other hand, serve to catalyze legislation that could harm all agriculture without necessarily helping the animals.

# 7 The Poultry Industry

The chicken and egg industries are, in many ways, the paradigm cases of intensive, industrialized agriculture. These industries represent far and away the largest numbers of animals used by humans—an estimated nine to ten billion worldwide. For this reason, argue Andrew Fraser and D. M. Broom, "if there are widespread welfare problems in this species, ... then a majority of the animals in the world which suffer because of man's activities are chickens."[1] The egg industry is also the most vertically integrated and mechanized of all animal agriculture and the oldest of confinement systems. A 1933 book on the industry describes battery egg cages and also cages for producing broilers.[2] (Broilers are not cage-raised today.) Laying hens are described as "egg machines,"[3] and the key concept of confinement for broilers is clearly articulated: "When poultry is prevented from taking exercise and fed an abundant and fat-forming ration, ... the birds not only gain in weight and in quality of flesh, but they actually produce a greater proportion of edible meat."[4] The book goes on to describe batteries as "poultry hotels" and asserts that the birds are "comfortable and happy."[5]

Thus, even at that early stage of development of the industry, the authors felt it necessary to justify the humaneness of confinement systems. In the 1960s, as books such as Ruth Harrison's *Animal Machines*[6] appeared in Britain and numerous articles began to react to confinement agriculture all over Europe, the battery cage for hens was seen as the exemplification of confinement. More welfare research has been carried out in Europe on the laying hen than on any other farm animal.[7]

In the United States, confinement production of chickens and eggs has not yet received the same level of attention in terms of welfare issues. Nonetheless, Frank Perdue, one of the nation's largest confinement broiler producers, for many years ran advertisements asserting that his company raised "happy chickens" and showing the animals living under pastoral, barnyard conditions. Undoubtedly, Perdue realized that confinement conditions would make the public uneasy. Indeed, in most areas of the country, one finds a market for "free-range" eggs and poultry.

According to Fraser and Broom, and contrary to what one sometimes hears from the industry, "There are few differences in behavior between the wild Burmese red jungle fowl *(Gallus gallus spadiceus)* and the domestic form *(Gallus gallus domesticus)*."[8] Furthermore, again contrary to what one may hear from the industry, chickens are not mindless, simple automata but are complex behaviorally, do quite well in learning, show a rich social organization, and have a diverse repertoire of calls. Anyone who has kept barnyard chickens also recognizes their significant differences in personality.

Unlike the swine industry, the U.S. chicken and egg industries have tended to "play ostrich" on welfare issues occasioned by their industry, adopting an "ignore it and hope it will go away" posture. It seems likely that the industry has felt that the public will not express a great deal of concern for chickens, perhaps seeing them as interchangeable clones. Perhaps, too, given the low price of eggs and chicken, once a luxury meat, the industry may believe that the public will not, as it were, bite the hand that feeds it.

Although it is certainly true that chickens will not generate the same sort of instantaneous response that calves do, it is myopic and self-deluding to think that public concern for the welfare of chickens is nonexistent. As Frank Perdue understood, there are few more vivid and classic bucolic images than chickens pecking contentedly in a barnyard; clever media manipulation could further tap our childhood memories of the story of The Little Red Hen. Conversely, few images in agriculture are more grating to common sense than chickens squeezed into small cages. To its credit, the Canadian egg industry has long recognized this potential and has funded research into alternative methods of egg production. One official of the Ontario Egg Board told me: "We are not wedded to any system of production. If the public wants greater attention to hen welfare, we are happy to oblige, as long as they are willing to pay for it."[9]

Given the U.S. poultry industry's hitherto cavalier treatment of welfare issues, I believe that it would be prudent for USDA to gather and analyze the extensive data amassed in Europe and Canada on welfare issues in egg and poultry production. In particular, the many alternative approaches to battery caging of hens developed in other countries should be force-fed into industry thinking.

## Welfare Issues in Battery-Cage Egg Production

In 1933, the average yield per hen was 70 eggs a year. A

yield of 150 eggs from a six-pound hen was considered unattainable.[10] Today a four-pound hen produces 275 eggs per year.[11] This increase is a result of improvements in genetics, nutrition, and disease control and, in no small measure, industrialization and intensive confinement systems. Productivity has increased without necessarily ensuring welfare, however. Although, for example, it has long been known that the stocking of fewer birds per cage leads to greater production per bird, it is nonetheless more economically efficient to put a greater number of birds into each cage, accepting lower productivity per bird but greater productivity per cage.[12] In other words, though each hen is less productive when crowded, the operation as a whole makes more money with a high stocking density: chickens are cheap, cages are expensive.

## Debeaking and Toe Trimming

The crowding of caged birds, up to six in a cage, has led to significant welfare issues. In the first place, hens in cages cannot establish normal social relationships, cannot behave as they have evolved to behave, and cannot escape from more aggressive animals. As a result, the system encourages the development of cannibalism and feather-pecking, which are costly in terms of both economics and welfare. The exact causes of these behaviors have not been determined,[13] but various factors have been implicated in their genesis, including high light intensities, housing systems, group size, nutrition, and hormonal factors.[14] These behaviors appear in chickens under extensive conditions but, where chickens can escape, do not cause the same degree of problems. Cannibalism can lead to high rates of mortality in battery chickens, and feather-pecking causes injury and loss of thermoregulatory ability. Though beak trimming, as practiced by the industry in both egg and broiler production, does not decrease the incidence of these behaviors, it does render the beak less effective in producing injury.[15]

For many years, the industry argued that beak trimming was a benign procedure, analogous to cutting nails in humans. However, it is now clear that this is not the case and that trimming causes behavioral and neurophysiological changes betokening both acute and chronic pain.

After hot-blade trimming, damaged nerves develop into extensive neuromas, known to be painful in humans and animals.[16] Furthermore, these neuromas show abnormal discharge and response patterns indicative of acute and chronic pain syndromes in mammals.[17] Behavioral and white-cell responses to beak trimming confirm this conclusion. There is also evidence that the pain of debeaking may ramify in pain in eating, weight loss, and "starve-out" in chicks.[18]

Obviously, then, beak trimming represents a major welfare issue. If the industry does not alter the systems that make it necessary, research should be undertaken to develop alternative methods of blunting the effect of the beak.

Laser trimming, new to the industry, should be looked at in terms of neuroma and chronic pain production.

In any case, it is clear that society will probably not accept the mutilation of the hens in a manner that produces chronic pain as a way of managing a "vice" stemming from a system that violates the animals' natures. A search for alternatives should be a top priority. Paul Siegel has argued that certain strains of chicken do not require debeaking, so perhaps the problem can be solved genetically.[19] M. W. Fox suggests that proper nutrition and lighting could also help control cannibalism.[20]

Toe trimming is also performed on laying hens to decrease claw-related injury. Research into whether or not this produces chronic pain is needed, as is research into alternatives.

### Behavioral Problems

Virtually all aspects of hen behavior are thwarted by battery cages: social behavior, nesting behavior, the ability to move and flap wings, dustbathing, space requirements, scratching for food, exercise, pecking at objects on the ground. D. G. M. Wood-Gush provides a detailed account of the discrepancy between chicken behavior under extensive conditions and that possible in confinement.[21] Hens typically live for about 72 weeks in such cages before they are shipped to slaughter.

### Exercise

The most obvious problem is lack of exercise and natural movement.[22] Under free-range conditions, hens walk a great deal. Wing flapping, which is common in free-range animals, is also prevented in cages. Comfort behavior is likewise truncated, as is leg stretching and preening.[23] Research has confirmed what common sense already knew—animals built to move must move. Studies have observed the animals' behavior in open conditions after long periods of deprivation. After being in a battery cage, hens show much wing flapping, and the longer they are caged, the more they flap.[24]

Lack of exercise has serious effects on bones and muscles. Caged birds have greater incidence of lameness, bone brittleness, osteoporosis, and muscle weakness than uncaged ones. Most significant, battery hens have a much higher incidence of broken bones than animals free to move.[25] H. B. Simonsen reported that 0.5 percent of free-range hens had broken wing bones at slaughter, in contrast to 6.5 percent of caged hens.[26] Fraser and Broom cite research showing that 29 percent of hens had broken bones before stunning at slaughter.[27]Obviously, giving hens the opportunity to move and exercise is a top research priority.

## Nesting

Nesting behavior is a primary activity of hens. According to Mench:

> Prior to egg-laying, feral or extensively housed fowl exhibit a characteristic sequence of behaviors associated with nest site selection. A period of restlessness and vocalization (pre-laying calls or "Gackeln") occurs which is followed by examination by the hen of potential nesting sites. When a nest site is finally selected, the hen performs rudimentary nest-building movements; oviposition occurs at a variable period of time following these behaviors. The most desirable nest site appears to be one which provides concealment and separation from conspecifics, and also protects on-going nesting and incubation behaviors from disturbance.[28]

Battery cages clearly cannot satisfy these needs, and this is the one area where behavioral signs of frustration are seen.[29] Hens housed in such cages display agitated pacing and escape behaviors that last two to four hours before oviposition.[30] Mench points out that the pacing is similar to the stereotyped pacing hens exhibit when they are thwarted in feeding behavior.[31]

Mench notes that hen demand for nests before laying is inelastic, with the animals willing to work to gain access to them and to suffer food and water deprivation in exchange for access. Building nests out of litter is also important to the hens; they choose building nests over using premolded ones and show greater frustration when given the premolded type.[32]

## Dustbathing

Mench has also surveyed the issue of depriving hens of the ability to dustbathe:

> On average, hens provided with loose material will perform dustbathing behaviors every other day, with each bout lasting approximately thirty minutes. The primary function of dustbathing appears to be to remove excess oil from the feathers and maintain them in a "fluffy" condition. Caged hens having no access to litter show dustbathing behavior as a vacuum activity. In addition, levels of both exploratory activity and dustbathing behavior increase in hens subjected to a period of litter deprivation. The performance of these vacuum and rebound activities suggests that hens have a motivation to dustbathe even when the appropriate external stimulus, litter, is absent in the environment.
>
> Preference tests appear to support this conclusion. Hens show a preference for cages with litter rather than wire floors when they are required to remain in the chosen cage for several hours. Hens will also enter a non-preferred small cage in order to have access to litter.[33]

Mench points out that many aspects of dustbathing are not clear, for example, the role of previous experience, the optimal and preferred type of substrate, and the role of social context. Furthermore, preference research has shown that material for dustbathing is not perceived by the animal as an absolute necessity, like food.[34] Research money could certainly be expended to clarify our understanding of this aspect of hen behavior. I believe that the money would be better spent on designing systems that meet the need, however.

## Social Behavior

Research indicates that social behavior in the domestic chicken under open conditions is similar to that of Burmese jungle fowl.[35] That research has been supplemented by studies of chickens gone feral for more than one hundred years and by studies of chickens deliberately released into the wild.[36] Ronald Kilgour has summarized the results of all this work:

> Behavior studies of wild jungle fowl of South East Asia have highlighted the birds' daily cyclical activity pattern of roosting, feeding, drinking and nesting with omnivorous feeding habits and secretive wary movement patterns. Hens were found in association with cocks, the hens' territory being about 1 ha and the cocks' about 5 ha.
>
> Studies of hens in a population that had been feral for about 100 years showed the following main features:
>
> —The birds established roosts, about 60 m apart and with 6–30 birds/roost and 1 harem/roost.
> —The amount of crowing by the males was related to status with the most crowing by the subordinate males. The dominant male acted as a suppressant to all hen fighting in his group.
> —The hens nested within 45 m of water but when broody only left the nest for a short period each day.
> —The broody hen and her chicks kept to themselves and threatened other hens that came within 6 m.
> —Chicks start to be left by the dam at 5–6 weeks when she returned to roost in a tree. At 10–12 weeks when chicks were feathered, the hen started to threaten them.
> —Chicks run ahead of the hen before weaning but behind her thereafter.
> —At 16–18 weeks, the brood breaks up and adult behavior patterns begin.

A study in Scotland compared the behavior of a group of hens released into the wild with a group fenced off and given some domestic care. Information on nest selection, laying, brooding, care of young, feeding and movement was collected. The work highlights the importance of the strong maternal behavior of the hen toward her spring-hatched chickens, walking over 3 km/day, walking with them 24 percent of the time. Their active working day lasted 16 hours and the hen initiated most of the behavior, especially feeding, tidbiting, pecking and scratching the ground. She also prevented fights between chicks. The importance of the male in organizing a harem and preventing fighting was also shown and confirmed the earlier research findings. The removal of the broody hen, the male and total confinement, key features of modern poultry farming, mean that behavior problems like severe pecking were bound to arise.[37]

All this behavior indicates the lack of fit between caged layers and their natural social predilections, as well as a similar lack of fit in broiler production. The precise nature of the friction between social preferences and caged layers has not yet been studied, however. This is a research issue with practical consequences, since such information can help guide the design and construction of rational alternative systems.

B. O. Hughes found that if hens were given a choice of feeding near cages containing zero to five unfamiliar birds, the hens preferred being near the empty cage, and the least preferred was the cage with the most birds.[38] If the other birds were not strangers, however, the hens preferred to be near them. Furthermore, hens prefer to be around other hens when they perform comfort behaviors, when laying eggs, and when feeding. This area needs further research.[39]

## Space

Along with exercise and movement, space is probably the area where the general public would see the greatest problem with the egg industry. The visual impact of hens squeezed together is stunning and evokes familiar, unfriendly metaphors of prisons and concentration camps.

When spatial requirements have been created for animals, for example, by USDA regulations for laboratory animals, they have been somewhat arbitrary and have satisfied no one—animal advocates still see the enclosures as cages, and scientists see the regulations as silly and unfounded. In order to rectify this situation, the functional dimension of space for the animals should be analyzed as a basis for rational modification of extant systems, as Alex Stolba did for swine (discussed in Chapter 4). Animals can languish in what appears to us to be large enclosures and do well in smaller ones. The operative principle here (discussed in Part 1) is Hal Markowitz's notion that an animal is a package of powers.

Daniel Rosenberg has described the sense in which primate housing is not enriched by large space alone.[40] He points out that two compatible macaques will be happier together in a small cage than if each was in a large cage, because they can engage in extensive social interactions. Similarly, providing chickens with additional *vertical* space containing perches might well benefit the animals more than enlarging the floor space. It is known that hens will use perches if they are supplied and prefer high perches to low ones. In addition, perches strengthen legs and reduce stress.[41]

On the other hand, certain minimal space requirements are evidently necessary for welfare. Again, common sense would not likely accept the notion that animals with bones and muscles do not need room to move. Thus research in this area should concentrate on identifying the multiple functions of space for the animal and how they can be accommodated in a cost-effective manner.

Mench discusses some research relevant to functional space.[42] She cites the work of M. S. Dawkins and S. Hardie,[43] which showed that the space needed by hens to perform comfort behaviors varied from 893 to 1,876 square centimeters; in groups, hens "squashed" together in performing the behaviors. Mench also describes research showing that

> hens housed in cages of different heights and areas show differences in their behavioral repertoire, with height affecting the rates of head stretching, body shaking, head scratching, feeding, drinking, cage pecking, and sitting, while area affects rates of head scratching, feather raising, drinking and cage pecking.[44]

Different cage configurations thus appear to provide outlets for different behaviors.

Even if battery cages are abandoned in favor of alternative systems that allow the animals greater space, it is useful to understand the ways in which such space should be designed. We saw earlier that in swine, escape areas are valuable to the animals; perches are similarly worthwhile for chickens. Space utilization by chickens is known to be influenced by group size, social relationships (i.e., familiarity or nonfamiliarity with other birds), social status, behavior that tends to be done in groups (feeding with familiar animals) rather than individually, and so on. Mench has reviewed research in this area.[45] Such knowledge can facilitate the development of animal-friendly systems for hens and can help refine the simplistic tendency to think that bigger is better.

## Boredom

It is easier to see the issue of boredom as a welfare problem for animals such as monkeys or swine, which are perceived as "intelligent," than for chickens. Nonetheless, there is good reason to believe that chickens can indeed get bored. Ingenious experiments by I. J. H. Duncan and B. O. Hughes have shown that, given a choice, hens will work for food rewards rather than just eat *ad libitum* even when food is provided.[46] Such results seem to force the conclusion that working alleviates boredom. H. J. Blokhuis suggests that feather pecking occurs in cages because the animals do not have enough normal stimulants at which to peck.[47] Research by M. C. Appleby and colleagues shows that laying hens in open conditions spend up to 16 percent of their time in nonforaging locomotion.[48] These findings accord well with our view that an animal is a bundle of evolved powers and that the inability to exercise those powers leads to frustration and boredom. Further research could well elucidate ways of enriching hen cages to alleviate boredom, as has been done in primate caging,[49] and perhaps thereby limit stress, "vices," and other pernicious consequences of current systems. Such enrichment could quickly pay for itself.

## Forced Molting

Egg laying is cyclical. The ovary becomes less active, and the diminution of sex hormones leads to new feather growth, which forces out the old feathers. At the end of this rest period, when feather regrowth is complete, the laying cycle resumes. But waiting for the cycle to proceed naturally is not cost-effective, since quantity and quality of eggs diminish, so producers have learned to induce molting.[50] This requires subjecting the animals to a sufficient stressor to inhibit ovulation. (Stress can inhibit reproductive capacity in all animals.) Producers accomplish this by withholding food and water, which is a significant stressor for the birds, since it is known that the demand for food and water is "inelastic," or fundamental.[51]

The standard forced molting protocol involves removal of food for up to twelve days and water deprivation for up to three days. Obviously, such an intentional stressor is quite traumatic for the animals, given the strength of the need for food and especially for water. In addition, the protocol usually involves withdrawal of daylight, another stressor to which the animals are unaccustomed. Indeed, so significantly adverse to welfare is this approach to artificial manipulation of the egg cycle that the British codes of practice since 1987 categorically recommend against using it.[52]

At the same time, according to Mench, "There are few studies on the effects of induced molting with regard to welfare."[53] Here, clearly, is a significant research issue. In particular, there is a need to investigate alternative protocols for inducing forced molts. The use of low-sodium diets[54] or low-calcium diets[55] is another protocol for inducing molting, and these too, need to be studied in terms of welfare. The development of methods of inducing molting that do not have adverse welfare effects should be made a high research priority.

## Wire Floors

Wire floors inhibit the ability of hens to dustbathe and to scratch and also violate their known preference for litter before and during oviposition.[56] Wire can also be responsible for soring and injury of feet and legs.[57] If hens continue to be raised in cages, research into animal-friendly flooring must be done.

## Cage Injuries

Battery cages are responsible for a variety of injuries, as birds are sometimes trapped in cages by the head and neck, body and wings, toes and claws, or other areas.[58] In addition, steep floors can cause foot deformities, and wire mesh can lead to feather wear.

## Attention to Individuals

Although battery cages theoretically allow for close monitoring of each bird, in reality the way cages are stacked, the periods of semidarkness, and the sheer numbers militate against close scrutiny. These factors lead to situations analogous to the case of the sow with a broken leg we discussed earlier. Research into improving monitoring could go a long way toward diminishing suffering. Care for individual animals, beyond viewing them as "expected losses" or "write-offs," is essential if public concerns about intensive agriculture are to be met.

# Improving Hen Welfare

There are three possible ways to improve the welfare of laying hens in battery systems: change the animal, modify the cage, or develop an alternative system.

## Changing the Animal

For many years, chicken producers have argued that the modern hen has been adapted, by natural and artificial selection, to the battery caging system. Our discussion thus far has shown that this is not the case, since breeders have looked at productivity, not specifically at welfare. There is no reason, however, that such breeding could not be done, given the rapidity with which chickens reproduce. Indeed, one reason genetic engineering is not being seriously considered in the poultry industry is that traditional genetics works so well.[59]

As mentioned earlier, certain strains of chickens seem to have less tendency toward cannibalism, pecking at other birds, and feather pecking.[60] Further research into incorporating these traits into commercial flocks should be a priority. Similarly, research into the genetic bases of lower reactivity to stressful situations could help create animals for which battery living was not a major concern or which even preferred it. The claim of better welfare would, of course, need to be confirmed by careful research.

On the other hand, such a strategy should be carefully monitored in terms of public acceptability. Though some animal welfare advocates see nothing wrong with using breeding or genetic engineering to create mindless farm animals that cannot suffer (to take an extreme example), that has to be a reflective opinion.[61] The public might well equate such work with "Frankenstein" activity. That is likelier to occur with genetic engineering than with breeding, however, especially if the selection is behavioral, not obviously somatically phenotypic.

An alternative approach to changing the animal is chemical. Mench describes this possibility:

> As our understanding of the neurochemistry and neurophysiology of fowl increases, it should also be possible to manipulate behavioral and physiological aspects of stress (and underlying emotional states themselves) by administering drugs, receptor agonists and antagonists, or precursors of neurochemicals. For example, the elevated aggression seen in feed-restricted birds during development can be decreased by increasing the dietary level of tryptophan, which is the precursor of serotonin. Serotonin probably not only affects aggression directly, but also has indirect effects because it decreases feeding motivation and thus a part of the stress associated with restriction.[62]

Like genetic engineering, such work could improve the well-being of animals. But again, public acceptability should be carefully considered. In an age of abhorrence of "chemicals," of exultation of the "natural," and of almost neurotic concern with food safety, such a strategy may end up doing more harm than good or substituting a new set of problems for old ones.

## Cage Modification

If caging systems are to continue, at least in the short run, it is essential to make them animal-friendly. Cage modification research and design should take into account the needs of hens we have discussed.

The modified cage should

1. Accommodate the hen's nesting requirements.
2. Guard against the injuries described earlier.
3. Minimize discomfort.

4. Allow birds, as far as possible, to express their natural behaviors.
5. Probably have perches.
6. Allow for ways to alleviate boredom.
7. Allow for less crowding and more animal-friendly stocking density.
8. Allow for movement and exercise.

Clearly, deciding which behavioral needs to meet, how much space to allow the birds, how much exercise, how much alleviation of boredom, and so on is going to be not a purely scientific task but rather one in which science engages the social ethic and economic reality. In my view, research into cage design should at least take cognizance of all the considerations we have discussed. Obviously, some modifications are much easier and cheaper than others—designing a cage with perches or nesting boxes or vertical space is a lot easier than designing one that meets social or exercise needs.

Fraser and Broom cite the "getaway" cage as an example of an alternative system (Figure 7.1).[63] They describe it and its problems as follows:

> These cages house about twenty hens on two levels and they have nests, perches and a sand bathing area. The design of get-away cages developed so far poses practical problems because of the large number of cracked and dirty eggs and the difficulties of egg collection. Welfare problems exist for those few individuals which fail to find the water nipples or which are attacked by other birds. Inspection of the birds is quite often difficult so these problems may not be readily discovered.[64]

## Alternative Systems

Perhaps the most prima facie plausible response to concern about cages is eliminating them in favor of something else. A much modified, ethologically based, animal-friendly cage is still a cage. In this area, agriculture can perhaps be guided by the zoo experience; increasing numbers of zoos are, wherever possible, moving away from cages to open areas with moats. A great deal of work on such alternative systems for hens is being done in Europe in the face of legislation and regulation. A major research priority should be a review by competent scientists of this literature and such systems for economic and production viability in the United States. We should piggyback on European work, not reinvent the wheel.

The main alternative approaches that have been developed in Europe are deep litter systems, percheries, straw yards, and aviaries.

### Deep Litter

Deep litter systems were quite widely used in Europe in the 1960s. The

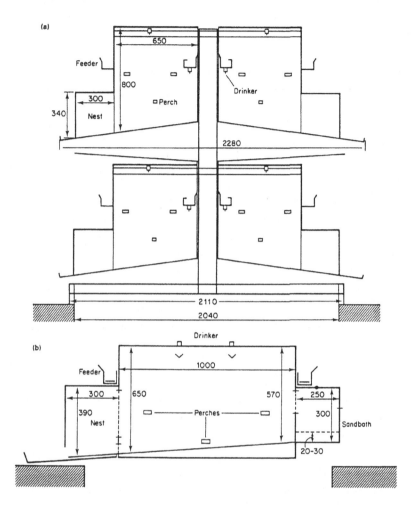

**Figure 7.1.** Section diagrams of two forms of getaway cages (dimensions in mm). (a) Getaway cage with rollaway nest. (b) Getaway cage with rollaway nest and sandbath. From A. F. Fraser and D. M. Broom, *Farm Animal Behaviour and Welfare* (London: Baillière Tindall), 1990, p. 379.

birds are housed entirely indoors with at least part of the floor covered in deep litter, such as wood shavings. Part of the floor may be slatted over a pit to collect droppings. Nest boxes are provided and accessed from corridors for easy egg collection, or floors are sloped to allow mechanical egg collection. The birds are free to move around, mingle, and exercise.[65] Problems include fighting and the extra difficulty in collecting eggs. Such a system is sometimes used for breeding flocks to facilitate natural matings.

### Percheries

A perchery is a modified deep litter system with perches provided.

### Covered Straw Yards

The covered straw yard, developed by David Sainsbury,[66] is claimed to be economically viable. It is basically a simple, uninsulated, naturally ventilated shed, deeply strawed. Each bird is given a space allowance of about 0.27 m$^2$, and the animals are provided with nest boxes, perches, hanging feeders, and waterers. Birds spend a good deal of time scratching, searching for food (grain is scattered in the straw), and dustbathing. Surprisingly, birds in straw yards performed as well as birds in cages:

> The result, which was most surprising, was that the food conversion efficiency was marginally better in the straw yard than in the cage-house. As the straw yard has other advantages, it is worthy of more consideration. The advantages are that running costs are generally low, there are no fans and a minimum of artificial lighting, and there is nothing mechanical to go wrong. Straw is converted into a valuable manure, the quality of the eggs is good, being comparable to eggs from birds in a cage system, but the straw eggs being richer in colour and richer in B$_{12}$. *There also appear to be no welfare problems.*
>
> It is interesting to speculate on the more efficient food conversion by chickens in the yard. It is noticeable that the birds are much better feathered in the yard, which probably improves their heat retention, and it is also found that they produce firmer droppings and spend less time in eating. It is possible that the caged bird eats and drinks more than it really requires because of the boredom of its existence, whilst straw yard birds spend time in activity on and in the litter and derive certain beneficial by-products from it. It should be noted, however, that the results for food consumption in straw yards found in my own studies have not been repeated by others, and further investigation is required on a wider scale to elucidate this finding.[67]

Sainsbury's summary of the performance of hens housed in covered straw yards from 20 to 72 weeks during 1984-85 is instructive. The food intake for the period was moderate (138 g/bird/day), while egg yield per hen was a satisfactory 282.8. Contrary to adverse expectations, only 1 percent of the eggs were recovered from the floor, and second-quality eggs amounted to 9.2 percent of the total production. Mortality was low (3.1 percent). Finally, the uninsulated, naturally ventilated shed maintained a mean temperature of 11.2° centigrade.[68]

### Aviaries

Many systems fall under the designation of aviary, which is essentially a conventional deep litter system with extra floors of wire or slats, each floor containing feeders, waterers, and nest boxes. Aviaries allow for far greater stocking density than is possible in simple deep litter houses, which in turn lowers the capital cost per bird, creates a warmer environment, and thereby reduces food consumption.[69] As a function of the warmer environment, greater ventilation is possible, which improves the drying of litter and eliminates condensation. According to Sainsbury "There is a widespread belief in both the research and commercial elements of the poultry industry that the aviary arrangement offers the best alternative for intensively housed birds which can be kept in controlled environment housing."[70]

Sainsbury examined the performance data for all the relevant alternative systems compared to battery cages and came up with interesting figures. The average egg yield per bird per annum was highest in battery cages (260) and lowest in free range (220). The deep litter and aviary systems (250 each) compared well with the battery system, while straw yard hens averaged 240 eggs in a year. The biggest difference between systems came in the number of birds per person. In battery cages one person could manage 10,000 hens; in aviaries 9,000; in deep litter 8,000; in straw yards 4,500; and in free range only 1,800. Food consumption per bird per annum varied little, differing by only 3 kg. The hearty eaters were free range birds (46 kg), deep litter birds ate least (42.5 kg). Birds in battery cages and those in aviaries ate the same amount (43 kg), which was slightly less than straw yard birds (45.5 kg). In total costs per bird there was little difference between battery cages (£9.16), deep litter (£9.36), and aviary (£9.36). Straw yard costs were a little higher (£10.21) and free range highest (£11.75).[71]

More recently, T. Tanaka and J. F. Hurnik compared both behavior and performance of laying hens housed in battery cages with that of hens housed in an aviary system. From a behavioral point of view,

> stereotyped behaviors occurred 5 to 10 times more in caged birds than in aviary birds. Comfort behaviors in caged birds were reduced to 14 to 19 percent of that recorded in aviary birds. ... The results of the present study indicate strongly that aviaries provide more freedom for movement and thus better opportunity for manifestation of comfort behaviors than battery cages *even when the cage housing density was lower than recommended for general commercial units* [three to a cage].[72]

At the same time, "the egg production ratio in the aviary was slightly lower than that in cages, but it was above the commercial level."[73] The data from Tanaka and Hurnik are shown in Table 7.1.

**Table 7.1. Production performance of caged and aviary hens**

| Measurement | Type of housing[a] | Age (weeks) 23 | 27 | 31 | 35 | 39 | 43 | 47 | 51 | 55 | 59 | 63 | x̄[b] |
|---|---|---|---|---|---|---|---|---|---|---|---|---|---|
| Daily feed consumption (g/bird) | C | 52.5 | 99.1 | 113.9 | 116.0 | 132.2 | 134.0 | 124.8 | 139.7 | 145.4 | 145.2 | 127.9 | 127.8 |
|  | A | 95.3 | 122.3 | 123.3 | 119.6 | 133.9 | 128.7 | 135.2 | 149.9 | 123.8 | 117.2 | 123.8 | 127.8 |
| Hen-day egg production (%) | C | 49.9 | 85.4 | 95.4 | 93.8 | 93.0 | 91.7 | 90.6 | 89.2 | 86.4 | 84.3 | 82.3 | 89.2 |
|  | A | 28.2 | 92.8 | 92.3 | 84.2 | 88.7 | 89.6 | 89.1 | 87.4 | 83.9 | 82.1 | 78.7 | 86.9 |
| Average egg weight (g) | C | 46.9 | 52.1 | 55.8 | 57.7 | 57.9 | 59.0 | 60.8 | 61.5 | 61.7 | 61.9 | 63.4 | 59.2 |
|  | A | 46.9 | 52.6 | 55.7 | 56.8 | 58.7 | 60.0 | 60.4 | 59.7 | 62.0 | 63.0 | 62.6 | 59.2 |
| Eggshell deformation (μm) | C | 26.2 | 24.7 | 23.8 | 24.3 | 22.9 | 24.3 | 25.6 | 25.7 | 26.4 | 27.2 | 27.0 | 25.2 |
|  | A | 25.3 | 26.1 | 23.6 | 24.5 | 23.6 | 25.4 | 26.0 | 26.8 | 27.1 | 27.7 | 26.8 | 25.8 |

Source: T. Tanaka and J. F. Hurnik, "Comparison of Behavior and Performance of Laying Hens Housed in Battery Cages and an Aviary," *Poultry Science* 71 (1992): 242. Reprinted with permission.

[a] C = battery cages; A = aviary. Mortality for C = 5.1% and for A = 5.9%.
[b] Mean values from 27 to 63 weeks.

Researching aviary systems for the U.S. industry, then, should be a top priority. Appleby et al. provide a good recent summary of alternative systems in relation to welfare.[74]

# Problems in Broiler Welfare

The broiler industry has attracted a good deal less public attention than the egg industry, and much less research into and discussion of broiler welfare has occurred.[75] Because of genetics, nutrition, and intensification, the modern broiler reaches market weight (1.5–2 kg) in 7 weeks, a reduction of nearly two-thirds from the time it took the traditional broiler.[76]

Broiler housing resembles the deep litter system for eggs. Birds are introduced at one day of age and kept together for 7 weeks in groups of ten thousand to twenty thousand; needless to say, the animals are very crowded by the end of this period.

### Inspection

Obviously, in the system described, it is going to be impossible to check on individual animals. Weak, sick, injured, or suffering animals are not detected. Down animals may be trampled. Once again, we have a problem of concern for individuals in large confinement operations. Research into alternative building design to help correct the situation would probably be a public-opinion priority.

### Problems of Fast Growth

With the breeding of broilers for fast growth and heavy musculature, little attention was paid to bone development and other areas under genetic control. The many diseases that have resulted must be considered a function of this approach to broiler production. They include leg weakness, ascites, sudden death or "flip-over," deep pectoral myopathy, and right ventricular hypertrophy.[77] Moreover, as Fraser points out, weak legs lead the birds to sit in soiled litter, which in turn produces breast blisters and hock burns, since the fecal material is corrosive.[78]

I. J. H. Duncan sees management of such problems as a primary candidate for research. He advocates research into short-term solutions as well as genetic selection to eliminate these concerns.[79]

### Food Restriction in Broiler Breeders

Duncan has eloquently stated the problem of food restriction: "Animal breeders will have to realize that they cannot proceed indefinitely to select for growth rate and appetite without running into problems with the breeding stock, which have to be maintained in a non-obese state."[80]As a result of such selection, broilers used for breeders must be kept under severe food restriction—they simply convert too efficiently. Since food is such a primordial, inelastic demand, it is likely these animals suffer. This problem should obviously be addressed.

Duncan suggests two possible short-term solutions that could be investigated: reducing nutrient density so the animals must spend more time feeding, and changing lighting schedules so more of the available light period is occupied with important maintenance behavior.[81]

### Space, Crowding, and Group Size

As Fraser and Broom point out, little is known of the effects of space limitation, crowding, and group size on welfare in broiler operations. These areas should be researched.[82]

### Alternative Systems

As far as I have been able to determine, there are virtually no other systems for broiler production, except for a small number of broilers raised under free-range conditions, and these have not been much studied. After the foundational research described above has been done, further research should be undertaken to design cost-effective broiler systems that avoid the problems we have discussed and provide for the animals' behavioral, social, and other needs in an animal-friendly fashion.

## Handling, Transportation, and Slaughter of Poultry

Although we take up the issues of handling, transportation, and slaughter last, they are by no means trivial. At the same time, they are probably easier to deal with than most of the issues already discussed.

### Destruction of Baby Male Chicks

Millions of newly hatched chicks are killed in the egg industry. They have been killed by suffocation in plastic bags, decapitation, carbon dioxide, and crushing. Carbon dioxide is purported to be the most humane of these methods.[83] Research is necessary into how the industry is killing these chicks and into ways of providing humane deaths for the baby birds.

## Handling, Capture, and Transportation

Fraser points out that "chickens are very much disturbed by close contact with people for man is a large and dangerous animal to a chicken."[84] Capture is thus highly stressful to chickens, both spent laying hens and broilers. Between 10 and 30 percent of broilers in Europe are injured during capture and transport, and 29 percent of spent hens have freshly broken bones (as mentioned earlier) by the time of preslaughter stunning.[85] These injuries are a function of bone weakness and rough handling. Hens are pulled from battery cages manually by the legs, carried by one leg in groups of two to five, and put into crates. Broilers are caught by catch gangs off the floors.

Both processes have been shown to result in physical and psychological trauma and stress. After all, these animals, which are unaccustomed to any human physical contact, are suddenly violently wrenched from the environment to which they are habituated. It is well known that breaking routine is stressful for animals, and that is certainly true here.[86]

Duncan has shown that some of this stress can be eliminated by using mechanical broiler catchers, which are driven through the broiler house and scoop up the broilers.[87] Research is needed to develop and refine such methods for hens and broilers.

Crating and transportation also need to be evaluated, since they too serve as major stressors for the birds. Once that is done, new animal-friendly trucking and crating can be studied. At the moment, most research that has been carried out on transportation is, according to Mench, difficult to interpret, "since many variables, including handling and crating, are confounded."[88]

## Slaughter

The issue of humane slaughter for poultry could benefit from research. As Mench points out, there is considerable debate over whether the electrical stunning currently used in poultry suffices to produce unconsciousness. It has been suggested that stunning voltages be raised to produce cardiac fibrillation.[89] The effect of such a change on bleed-out and carcass quality needs to be examined.

Mench notes that hypoxia holds promise as a commercial stunning method, using nitrogen or argon gas. The latter actually improved carcass quality.[90]

## Genetic Engineering

The poultry industry has not been quick to embrace genetic engineering, perhaps because conventional breeding proceeds so quickly in poultry. Some work has been done, however. Disease resistance has been successfully incorporated into poultry, with no adverse effects. On the other hand, experiments with increasing size have led to skeletal problems affecting welfare negatively. As with all other animals, genetically engineered modifications should be carefully assessed for welfare implications before the changes are introduced into the industry.

# 8 Reflections

A new social ethic for animals is emerging in the Western world, replacing the traditional emphasis on cruelty and kindness. This ethic grows out of a realization on the part of society that new uses of animals have developed in the mid-twentieth century which are significantly different from traditional, extensive, husbandry-based agriculture. In traditional agriculture, producers did well if and only if animals did well, thereby generating what I have called the ancient contract between humans and animals, epitomized in the western ranchers' dictum, "We take care of the animals; the animals take care of us." In addition, in traditional agriculture, one could not selectively care for parts of the animals' biological and psychological natures and ignore others. Successful animal agriculture was about placing animals in environments as congenial to them as possible and for which they had evolved, generating as little friction as possible, and then augmenting their natural coping ability with protection against predation, drought, and famine. The biblical shepherd leading his animals to green pastures provides a vivid paradigm.

In contradistinction to this pastoral picture, the twentieth century saw the advent of animal use that was much more patently exploitative. The rise of animal use in science for studying disease, trauma, wounds, and basic biological processes, and for toxicological testing did not fit the contract, for it did not provide benefits for the animals used. Even more important, the development of technological agriculture, based in the application of industrial methods to the raising of animals, represented animal use far removed from the ancient contract. Industry replaced husbandry—with the help of new technology, one could meet the select needs of animals that were relevant to efficiency and productivity without respecting the animals' entire telos or psychological and biological natures.

In an era of great concern about fairness in the treatment of the disenfranchised, occurring at roughly the same time as far-reaching changes in animal use, it was inevitable that the social moral searchlight would fall on the new agriculture. To evaluate the radical changes in animal use, society needed a new moral vocabulary with which to talk about animal suffering that was not the result of sadism or cruelty but simply an outgrowth of the attempt to produce cheap, plentiful food in a profitable way. Since moral concepts stem from previous moral concepts, society looked to its moral machinery for evaluating the social use of humans and applied it to animals, mutatis mutandis.

In democratic societies, the interests of individuals are protected from submersion beneath the common good by the notion of rights. Rights are moral/legal fences built around individuals to protect, even from the general welfare, their fundamental interests as dictated by their natures. And it is precisely this notion that mainstream social thought is exporting to animals, as evidenced by the new Swedish farm animal law. If modern agriculture no longer guarantees the respect for animals' natures presupposed in traditional agriculture, that role must be taken up by law and regulation. This is the sense in which animal rights is a mainstream notion for assessing animal treatment. It is, in essence, a vehicle for preserving the ancient contract in the face of radical change in animal use. By the same token, the agricultural community should understand that this concept of animal rights is not radically different from animal welfare but represents the form that animal welfare concerns are currently assuming.

In the face of this change in the social ethic, it is imperative that agriculture immediately address the welfare (or rights) issues occasioned by animal production systems and modify or replace them so as to make them animal-friendly. We have surveyed the major animal industries and, rather surprisingly, have found that there already exist viable alternative approaches to many of the most problematic aspects of current systems. (The semi-extensive systems for raising swine without gestation crates provide an excellent example.) For other areas, such as livestock transport, a relatively small expenditure of research money should produce noticeable results fairly quickly; the issues are, after all, nowhere near as complex as finding a cure for cancer or putting a man on the moon. We have furthermore seen that, in cases such as livestock transport or branding of cattle, solving the welfare issue goes hand in hand with improving economic gain. The greatest barrier to resolving the animal welfare problems in agriculture is the failure of the industry to see them as problems and an attendant mindset that suppresses ethical and valuational questions or redefines them in strictly economic terms.

In general, our society is plagued by a business management mindset that tends to define activities in quantitative terms of efficiency and productivity; aspects of a problem that do not lend themselves to such redefinition are ignored or discounted. Thus a high USDA official dismissively referred to western ranchers as "a bunch of goddamn romantics" because they were not exclusively focused on the bottom line—they also worried about their way of life, husbandry, and so on. The same cancer has eaten away at our institutions of higher learning. Universities are governed by "professional administrators" —bean-counters, not scholars—who count numbers of articles for tenure and promotion and numbers of students taught, and for whom qualitative notions are irrelevant if not incomprehensible.

In a personal vein, I recall one administrator approaching me and asking permission to videotape my courses and circulate the tapes around the state because "you are such a good teacher." "In this way," he continued, "you can reach thousands more people." He was amazed when I categorically refused. "Why?" he asked in astonishment. "Because I *am* such a good teacher," I replied. I encountered the same insensitivity from another administrator, who argued that I should double the enrollment in one of my classes. "You are doing such a great job with fifty," he warbled, "I'm sure you can do twice as well with a hundred!"

I am fearful of an approach to agriculture that uses only a "bottom line" yardstick. First of all, as I have said, qualitative distinctions are invisible to it. Second, intimately related and equally important, it tends to ignore costs (and benefits) that do not show up on a balance sheet. Yet the industrialization of agriculture has produced numerous hidden costs that mitigate its much-touted efficiency. One of those costs, the subject of this book, is animal suffering. Thus it is true that chicken has stayed at virtually the same low price for twenty years, but at the expense of the animals' well-being. But there are others worth reflecting on.

Another such cost is environmental. Industrialized animal agriculture, it is well known, is totally dependent on high inputs, specifically, on fossil fuel, a resource we now realize is limited. It also requires significant amounts of water. At the same time, disposal of enormous amounts of animal and agricultural wastes concentrated in a small area is a major problem, often resulting in groundwater contamination.

Yet another hidden cost of industrialized agriculture is the effect on rural communities and the agrarian way of life. Too few farmers realize that the same forces that put animals in boxes have put farmers in financial boxes. With capital inexorably replacing labor, smaller independent producers are simply not in a position to compete with large corporate entities that have unlimited resources. This in turn means that farmers go out of business, become mortgaged to the hilt, or become, in essence, contractual serfs to large corporations, as has occurred in the poultry business and in some portions of the swine industry. None of these alternatives is good for the agricultural way of life. Obviously, going out of business means the loss of one more family farm.

Chronic indebtedness leads to a highly stressful way of life and to farmers being forced to do anything required to survive—witness the case of the sow with a broken leg. Thus people who may strongly believe in the husbandry ethic are thus sometimes forced to violate it in order to survive. And finally, working for a large corporate operation erodes the independence historically characteristic of the agricultural way of life and must inevitably create a deep sense of instability.

Ironically, increasing numbers of urban and suburban citizens look to rural agricultural communities as an escape from urban blight—and thereby often further destroy the character of these communities, since the emigrés do not fit the traditional rural values but rather bring their urban values with them. They cannot in any case go into farming except in a hobby fashion unless they are independently wealthy; it is well known that young people simply cannot afford to become farmers. Many ranchers, even those who have inherited their operations, must work multiple jobs to keep the ranch afloat, often because urban people have moved into the area, demanding services that raise land values and taxes.

We can thus see that our apparently cheap food supply has a variety of interrelated hidden costs. We have already found that some alternatives to severe confinement of animals are viable and profitable—and semi-extensive. A move toward less intensiveness where possible in animal agriculture may go some of the way toward addressing these unstated costs.

Consider the case of swine. As we have seen, semi-extensive swine operations require less capitalization, less initial investment, and thus less overhead and input. By the same token, waste disposal is less of a problem, as the wastes are dispersed over a larger area. (In traditional extensive agriculture, animal wastes served to enhance pasture, and pasture served to sustain animals.) If the hog market is depressed, one can quickly convert the land to a cash crop with minimal loss. Since little capitalization is required, it is possible for people without vast resources to enter the business.

For such an operation to be successful, however, one needs "pig smart" labor and probably a proportionally larger labor force. Although this is a problem, it is also an opportunity. With more and more people looking for a healthier environment than the cities where they can live and raise a family, why not train people to own and/or work in such operations? Why not provide tax subsidies or incentives to people who are willing to enter into such a business and lure such employees? One of the standard justifications for intensification is the lack of a farm labor force and the high cost of labor. With people fleeing urban life and seeking a more "natural," rural existence, could not social subsidization of such semi-extensive agriculture, as occurs in Europe, solve a great many social problems? In a single stroke, one would be revitalizing rural communities with people who would be a part of those communities, not merely urban exiles hanging their hats; creating a more sustainable and environmentally sound agriculture; and resurrecting an agriculture of husbandry more closely allied to the ancient contract. Though there are, to my knowledge, no similar examples extant in the poultry industry, perhaps such systems could be developed there also, provided that society is willing to commit to that kind of change.

Obviously, my suggestion depends on society's providing a helping hand to such operations. But why not? Society has essentially paid for the development of industrialized agriculture through research at land-grant colleges and universities. In addition, if we are indeed concerned about rural communities, sustainability, environmental preservation, and fair treatment of animals, we should be prepared to pay for it. The percentage of disposable income we in the United States spend on food is the lowest in the world. Ought we not be prepared to put some of that bounty back to preserve the other values we have neglected or eroded in our rush to achieve that status? At the very least, the feasibility of this idea should be researched.

Animal agriculture is as old as civilization, and our ancient contract with animals, for all its flaws, has been a model of natural justice and fairness. We have, in most cases, coexisted with our domestic animals better than we have with one another. Their presence has been a manifest and positive one, reflected and extolled in our arts, crafts, literature, mythology, song, and story. Our children still sing of Old MacDonald's farm. No one sings of Old MacDonald's factory. We must do what needs to be done to preserve that ancient contract, else we diminish not only the animals but ourselves as well.

# Notes

## Chapter 1. The New Social Ethic for Animals

1. For a detailed discussion of the traditional anticruelty ethic, see Bernard E. Rollin, *Animal Rights and Human Morality,* 2nd edition (Buffalo, N.Y.: Prometheus Books, 1992), part II.

2. Ibid.

3. E.g., Henry Salt, *Animals' Rights: Considered in Relation to Social Progress* (Clark's Summit, Pa.: SAR, 1980), originally published in 1892; E. P. Evans, *Evolutional Ethics and Animal Psychology* (New York: Appleton, 1898).

4. A. N. Rowan, *Of Mice, Models, and Men* (Albany: SUNY Press, 1984), pp. 64–65.

5. R. E. Taylor, *Scientific Farm Animal Production* (New York: Macmillan, 1992), p. 6.

6. J. L. Meij, *Mechanization in Agriculture* (Chicago: Quadrangle Books, 1960), p. 65.

7. Taylor, *Scientific Farm Animal Production,* p. 6.

8. Thomas Wolfle, personal communication. 1990. Cf. National Research Council, *Recognition and Alleviation of Pain and Distress in Laboratory Animals* (Washington, D.C.: National Academy Press, 1992), p. 7.

9. B. E. Rollin, "An Ethicist's Commentary on the Case of the Sow with a Broken Leg Waiting to Farrow," *Canadian Veterinary Journal* 32 (October 1991).

10. Paul Thompson, "Ideals in Animal Agriculture" (paper delivered at the University of Maryland International Conference on Farm Animal Welfare, June 1991).

11. Ruth Harrison, *Animal Machines* (London: Vincent Stuart, 1964).

12. F. W. R. Brambell, *Report of the Technical Committee to Enquire into the Welfare of Animals Kept under Intensive Livestock Husbandry Systems* (London: HMSO, 1965).

13. Stanley Godlovitch, Roslind Godlovitch, and John Harris, *Animals, Men, and Morals* (New York: Grove Press, 1977).

14. *New York Times,* October 25, 1988: Swedish Farm Animals Get a Bill of Rights, p.1.

15. Andrew Rowan, "Animal Experimentation and Society: A Case Study of an Uneasy Interaction," in D. J. Roy, B. E. Wynne, R. W. Old (eds.), *Bioscience—Society* (New York: John Wiley, 1991), pp. 261–281.

16. Thomas Wolfle, personal communication. 1990.

17. See M. A. Fox, *The Case for Animal Experimentation: An Evolutionary and Ethical Perspective* (Berkley: University of California Press, 1986); M. A. Fox, "Animal Experimentation: A Philosopher's Changing Views," *Between the Species* 3(1987):55–60, 75, 80, 82. Michael A. Fox is Professor of Philosophy at Queens University in Ontario. He is often confused with Michael W. Fox, veterinarian and vice president at the Humane Society of the United States.

18. *Animal Legal Defense Fund v. The Department of Environment Conservation of the State of New York* (1985), Index #6670/85.

19. Rollin, *Animal Rights and Human Morality,* Part I.

20. Steve Suther, "Are You an Animal Rightist?" *Beef Today,* April 1993 (see also the sidebar comments by animal scientist R. Warner).

21. *Parents* magazine, *Parents Poll on Animal Rights, Attractiveness, Television, and Abortion* (New York: Kane and Parsons, 1989).

22. Charles McCarthy, Office of Protection from Research Risks, National Institutes of Health, personal communication. 1988.

23. *New York Times,* October 25, 1988.

24. Office of Technology Assessment, *New Developments in Biotechnology: Public Perceptions of Biotechnology* (Washington, D.C., 1987).

25. R. Jeffrey Smith, "NCI Bioassays Yield a Trail of Blunders," *Science* 204(1979):1287–1292.

26. Vernon Riley, "Mouse Mammary Tumors: Alteration of Incidence as Apparent Function of Stress," *Science* 189(1975):465–469.

27. M. B. Visscher, "Review of *Animal Rights and Human Morality,*" *New England Journal of Medicine* 306(1982):1303–1304.

28. *Animal Legal Defense Fund v. Madigan,* 791 F, Supp. 797 (D.D.C. 1992).

29. National Cattlemen's Association, *NCA Summary Report: Consumer Research on the Animal Care Issue,* Summer 1991.

30. A. N. Rowan, "Beefing about Farm Animal Production" (paper delivered at Alberta Feed Industry Animal Conference, Lethbridge, 1992.)

31. Joseph Stookey, personal communication. 1993.

32. Stanley Curtis, "Future Directions of Science and Public Policy" (paper delivered at the University of Maryland International Conference on Farm Animal Welfare, June 1991.)

33. Temple Grandin, "Cleaning House: Let's Be Proactive on Animal Care Issues," *National Cattleman,* August 1991, p. 26; Temple Grandin, "Proactive Activism," *Meat and Poultry,* August 1991, p. 29.

## Chapter 2. Welfare Research and Scientific Ideology

1. For a detailed account of points 2–4, see B. E. Rollin, *The Unheeded Cry: Animal Consciousness, Animal Pain, and Science* (Oxford: Oxford University Press, 1989).

2. American Veterinary Medical Association Executive Board Minutes, July 14–15, 1982, p. 11.

3. Council for Agricultural Science and Technology, *Scientific Aspects of the Welfare of Food Animals,* Report no. 91, November 1981, p. 1.

4. D. M. Broom, "The Scientific Assessment of Animal Welfare," *Applied Animal Behavior Science* 20(1988):5–19.

5. M. S. Dawkins, *Animal Suffering: The Science of Animal Welfare* (London: Chapman and Hall, 1980), preface and chapter 1; I. J. H. Duncan, "Animal Rights—Animal Welfare: A Scientist's Assessment," *Poultry Science* 60(1981):490.

6. B. E. Rollin, "On the Nature of Illness," *Man and Medicine* 4, 3(1979):157–172.

7. B. E. Rollin, "The Concept of Illness in Veterinary Medicine," *Journal of the American Veterinary Medical Association* 182(1983):122–125.

8. Rollin, *Unheeded Cry,* passim.

9. Ibid., chapter 5.

10. J. W. Mason, "A Re-evaluation of the Concept of 'Non-specificity' in Stress Theory," *Journal of Psychiatric Research* 9(1971):332–333.

11. See B. E. Rollin, "Some Ethical Concerns in Animal Research: Where Do We Go Next?"

in R. M. Baird and S. E. Rosenbaum (eds.), *Animal Experimentation: The Moral Issues* (Buffalo, N.Y.: Prometheus Books, 1991).

12. Rollin, *Unheeded Cry,* chapter 1.

13. W. T. Keeton and J. L. Gould, *Biological Science* (New York: W.W. Norton, 1986), p. 6.

14. Sylvia Mader, *Biology: Evolution, Diversity, and the Environment* (Dubuque, Iowa: W. E. Brown, 1987), p. 15.

15. *Michigan State News* (February 27, 1989), p. 8.

16. Jay Katz, "The Regulation of Human Experimentation in the United States," *IRB* 9,1(1987):1–6.

17. Rollin, *Unheeded Cry,* passim.

18. Ibid., chapter 4.

19. Ibid., p. 104.

20. L. A. Merillat, *Principles of Veterinary Surgery* (Chicago: Alexander Eger, 1906), p. 223.

21. R. L. Kitchell and H. H. Erickson (eds.), *Animal Pain: Perception and Alleviation* (Bethesda, Md.: American Physiological Society, 1985).

22. David Hume, *A Treatise of Human Nature* (1777), ed. L. A. Selby-Bigge (Oxford: Oxford University Press, 1963), p. 176; "Panel Report on the Colloquium on Recognition and Alleviation of Animal Pain and Distress," *Journal of the American Veterinary Medical Association* 191,10(1987):1186–1191.

23. B. E. Rollin, "Animal Pain, Scientific Ideology, and the Reappropriation of Common Sense," *Journal of the American Veterinary Medical Association* 191,10(1987):1222–1227.

24. Rollin, *Unheeded Cry,* pp. 252–254.

25. Robert Dantzer and P. Mormède, "Stress in Farm Animals: A Need for Re-evaluation," *Journal of Animal Science* 57(1983):6–18.

26. I. J. H. Duncan, "Animal Rights—Animal Welfare: A Scientist's Assessment," *Poultry Science* 60(1981):489–499; Rollin, *Animal Rights and Human Morality.*

27. J. M. Stookey and J. F. Patience, "High Technology in Production of Pork and Its Implications," in Jerome Martin (ed.), *High Technology and Animal Welfare* (Edmonton: University of Alberta, 1991), pp. 61–79.

28. Dawkins, *Animal Suffering,* preface and introduction.

29. Ibid., p. 2.

30. Françoise Wemelsfelder, "Boredom in Animals," in M. W. Fox and L. Mickley (eds.), *Advances in Animal Welfare Science* (The Hague: Martinus Nijhoff, 1984), pp. 1–21.

31. Marian S. Dawkins, "From an Animal's Point of View: Motivation, Fitness, and Animal Welfare," *Behavioral and Brain Sciences* 13(1990):1–9.

32. I. J. H. Duncan and D. G. M. Wood-Gush, "Frustration and Aggression in the Domestic Fowl," *Animal Behavior* 20(1971):444 ff.

33. Hal Markowitz, *Behavioral Enrichment in the Zoo* (New York: Van Nostrand Reinhold, 1982); Hal Markowitz and Scott Line, "The Need for Responsive Environments," in B. E. Rollin and M. L. Kesel (eds.), *The Experimental Animal in Biomedical Research,* volume 1 (Boca Raton, Fla.: CRC Press, 1990), chapter 10.

34. Charge to the panel, May 15–17, 1987.

35. Bernard E. Rollin, *The Frankenstein Syndrome: Ethical and Social Issues in the Genetic Engineering of Animals* (New York: Cambridge University Press, 1995).

36. Vernon Pursel et al., "Genetic Engineering of Livestock," *Science* 244(1989):1281–1288.

## Chapter 3. The Beef Industry

1. Jeremy Rifkin, *Beyond Beef: The Rise and Fall of the Cattle Culture* (New York: Dutton, 1992); John Robbins, *Diet for a New America* (Walpole, N.H.: Stillpoint, 1987).

2. These observations are based on my seminars to and conversations with more than five thousand ranchers in Colorado, Wyoming, Montana, Nebraska, Nevada, Alberta, British Columbia, Texas, and South Dakota.

3. Robert E. Taylor, *Beef Production and the Beef Industry: A Beef Producer's Perspective* (Minneapolis: Burgess, 1984), p. 173.

4. Tom Field, "Effects of Hot Iron Branding on Value of Cattle Hides," in National Cattlemen's Association, *The Final Report of the National Beef Quality Audit, 1991,* (Englewood, Colo.: NCA, 1992) p. 127.

5. A. L. Neumann, *Beef Cattle,* 7th edition (New York: John Wiley, 1977), p. 311; Frank H. Baker (ed.), *Beef Cattle Science Handbook,* volume 19 (Boulder, Colo.: Westview, 1983), p. 422.

6. D. C. Lay et al., "Behavioral and Physiological Effects of Freeze or Hot-iron Branding on Crossbred Cattle," *Journal of Animal Science* 70(1992):330–336.

7. Gary L. Minish and Dan G. Fox, *Beef Production and Management* (Reston, Va.: Reston, 1979), pp. 111–112.

8. Unpublished research viewed by the author.

9. M. Georges et al., "On the Use of DNA Fingerprints for Linkage Studies in Cattle," *Genomics* 6(1990):461–474.

10. B. E. Rollin, "Pain, Paradox, and Value," *Bioethics* 3(1989):211–226.

11. Temple Grandin, "Handling and Slaughter of Livestock," in *CAST Task Force Welfare Report,* forthcoming.

12. Unpublished research.

13. R. M. Wuther, *South Dakota Farm and Home Research* 9(1958):16–19.

14. M. E. Ensminger, *Beef Cattle Science* (Danville, Ill.: Interstate, 1968), p. 407.

15. George Seidel, personal communication, September 1992.

16. Press release, Colorado State University, January 15, 1993.

17. *Report of the Animal Care Work Group to the NCA Animal Health Committee,* January 1992, p. 5.

18. Robert Mortimer, personal communication, 1991.

19. John Edwards, personal communication, 1987.

20. Grandin, "Handling and Slaughter of Livestock," p. 4.

21. Ibid., p. 5.

22. Temple Grandin, "Double Rail Restrainer Conveyor for Livestock Handling," *Journal of Agricultural Engineering Research* 41(1988):327–338; L. M. Panepinto, "A Comfortable Minimum Stress Method of Restraint for Yucatan Miniature Swine," *Laboratory Animal Science* 33(1983):95–97.

23. Grandin, "Handling and Slaughter of Livestock," p. 5.

24. Neumann, *Beef Cattle,* p. 337.

25. *Report of the Animal Care Work Group,* p. 7.

26. Ronald Kilgour, "The Application of Animal Behavior and the Humane Care of Farm Animals," *Journal of Animal Science* 46(1978):1478–1486.

27. Grandin, "Handling and Slaughter of Livestock," p. 12.

28. Neumann, *Beef Cattle,* p. 338.

29. John Archer, *Animals under Stress* (Baltimore: University Park Press, 1979).

30. Grandin, "Handling and Slaughter of Livestock," pp. 5–6.

31. *Report of the Animal Care Work Group,* p. 6.

32. C. C. Daly et al., "Cortical Function in Cattle during Slaughter: Conventional Captive Bolt Stunning Followed by Exsanguination Compared with Schechita Slaughter," *Veterinary Record* 122(1988):325–329.

33. J. M. Regenstein and Temple Grandin, "Religious Slaughter and Animal Welfare: An Introduction for Animal Scientists," in *Proceedings of the Annual Reciprocal Meats Conference,*

*American Meat Science Association* (Chicago: National Livestock and Meat Board, 1993), pp. 155–159.

34. Temple Grandin, "Humanitarian Aspects of *Shehitah* in the United States," *Judaism* 39(1990):436–446.

35. Jeffrey Rushen, "Aversion of Sheep to Handling Treatments, Paired Choice Studies," *Applied Animal Behavior Science* 16(1986):363–370.

36. Regenstein and Grandin, *Religious Slaughter,* p. 7.

37. D. F. Walker and J. T. Vaughn, *Bovine and Equine Urogenital Surgery* (Philadelphia: Lea and Febiger, 1980), pp. 27–37.

## Chapter 4. The Swine Industry

1. Ronald Kilgour and Clive Dalton, *Livestock Behavior: A Practical Guide* (Boulder, Colo.: Westview, 1984), p. 150.

2. Jim Mason and Peter Singer, *Animal Factories,* revised edition (New York: Harmony Books, 1990), p. 7.

3. Kilgour and Dalton, *Livestock Behavior,* p. 187.

4. Andrew Fraser and D. M. Broom, *Farm Animal Behaviour and Welfare,* 3d edition (London: Baillière Tindall, 1990), p. 305.

5. Kilgour and Dalton, *Livestock Behavior,* p. 187.

6. D. G. M. Wood-Gush, *Elements of Ethology* (London: Chapman and Hall, 1983), p. 38.

7. Temple Grandin, unpublished observations at the University of Illinois, personal communication. 1992.

8. Alex Stolba, "A Family System of Pig Housing, in *Alternatives to Intensive Husbandry Systems* (Potters Bar, Hertsfordshire, England: UFAW 1981), pp. 52–68. See also the discussion in Wood-Gush, *Elements of Ethology,* and D. G. M. Wood-Gush and Alex Stolba, "Behavior of Pigs and the Design of a New Housing System," *Applied Animal Ethology* 8(1981):583–585.

9. Wood-Gush and Stolba, "Behavior of Pigs."

10. Wood-Gush, *Elements of Ethology,* p. 196.

11. Wood-Gush and Stolba, "Behavior of Pigs," p. 584.

12. Wood-Gush, *Elements of Ethology,* p. 197.

13. Ibid.

14. C. Clanton, "Animal Welfare: Lessons from Europe," *National Hog Farmer,* December 15, 1990, p. 62.

15. Joseph M. Stookey, letter to Rick Klassen and Laurie Connor, February 16, 1993.

16. Ibid.

17. National Pork Producers Council, *Swine Care Handbook* (Des Moines, Iowa, 1992), p. 13.

18. B. E. Rollin, *Animal Rights and Human Morality,* 2d edition (Buffalo, N.Y.: Prometheus Books, 1992).

19. Kilgour and Dalton, *Livestock Behavior,* p. 187.

20. "Can Animals Think?" *Time* magazine, March 22, 1993, cover story.

21. Françoise Wemelsfelder, "Boredom and Laboratory Animal Welfare," in B. E. Rollin and M. L. Kesel (eds.), *The Experimental Animal in Biomedical Research,* Volume I (Boca Raton, Fla.: CRC Press, 1990).

22. B. E. Rollin, *The Unheeded Cry: Animal Consciousness, Animal Pain, and Science* (Oxford: Oxford University Press, 1989).

23. See the numerous discussions in W. Sybesma (ed.), *The Welfare of Pigs* (The Hague: Martinus Nijhoff, 1981).

24. Stookey, letter to Klassen and Connor.

25. Fraser and Broom, *Farm Animal Behaviour,* p. 363.

26. Stolba, "Family System."

27. Clanton, "Animal Welfare."

28. Wood-Gush, *Elements of Ethology,* pp. 197–198.

29. Clanton, "Animal Welfare."

30. Ibid.

31. Ibid., p. 64.

32. Stolba, "Family System," p. 65.

33. Wood-Gush, *Elements of Ethology,* p. 198.

34. C. Pijoan et al., "Extensive Methods of Swine Production," in *Minnesota Swine Conference for Veterinarians* (College of Veterinary Medicine, University of Minnesota, 1990), pp. 269–279.

35. Ibid., p. 269.

36. J. R. Morris and J. F. Hurnik, "An Alternative Housing System for Sows," *Canadian Journal of Animal Science* 70(1990):957–961.

37. Ibid., p. 957.

38. Ibid., p. 958.

39. "Pigs on Dirt," *Large Animal Veterinarian,* February 1993, pp. 5–7.

40. Ibid., p. 5.

41. Ibid., p. 6.

42. Ibid.

43. M. W. Fox, *Farm Animals: Husbandry, Behavior, and Veterinary Practice* (Baltimore: University Park Press, 1984), p. 64.

44. Kilgour and Dalton, *Livestock Behavior,* p. 152.

45. J. M. Stookey and J. F. Patience, "High Technology in Production of Pork and Its Welfare Implications," in J. Martin (ed.), *High Technology and Animal Welfare* (Edmonton: University of Alberta, 1991), p. 67.

46. G. K. Vestergaard, "An Evaluation of Ethological Criteria and Methods in the Assessment of Well-Being in Sows," *Annales de Recherches Veterinaire* 15, 2(1984):227–235.

47. Stookey and Patience, "High Technology," p. 68.

48. Frank Hurnik, personal communication, 1993. See also Zhensheng Loh and Frank Hurnik, "Paired Circular Crates: An Ideal Alternative for Farrowing," *Misset Pigs,* November–December 1991, pp. 31–33.

49. Fraser and Broom, *Farm Animal Behaviour,* p. 366.

50. Summarized in ibid., p. 360.

51. L. Backstrom, "Environment and Animal Health in Piglet Production," *Acta Veterinaria Scandinavica,* supplement 41(1973), 1–240; See also Ekesbo 1980, quoted in Fox, *Farm Animals,* p. 66.

52. Fraser and Broom, *Farm Animal Behaviour,* p. 361.

53. Ibid., p. 362.

54. Ibid.

55. Kilgour and Dalton, *Livestock Behavior,* p. 187.

56. *Management of Welfare of Farm Animals: The UFAW Handbook,* 3d edition (London: Baillière Tindall, 1988), p. 167.

57. Fraser and Broom, *Farm Animal Behaviour,* p. 327.

58. Ibid., p. 328; M. J. Bryant, "The Social Environment: Behavior and Stress in Housed Livestock," *Veterinary Record* 90(1972):351–359.

59. Fraser and Broom, *Farm Animal Behaviour,* p. 328.

60. Ibid., p. 367.

61. Cited in Stookey and Patience, "High Technology," p. 69.

62. Fox, *Farm Animals,* p. 51.

63. Ibid., p. 53.

64. J. J. McGlone and S. E. Curtis, "Behavior and Performance of Weaning Pigs in Pens Equipped with Hide Areas," *Journal of Animal Science* 60(1985):20–24.

65. Fraser and Broom, *Farm Animal Behaviour,* p. 368.

66. B. E. Rollin, "Moral, Social, and Scientific Aspects of the Use of Swine in Research," in M. E. Tumbleson (ed.), *Swine in Biomedical Research,* volume 1 (New York: Plenum, 1986).

67. Paul Hemsworth, "The Influence of Handling by Humans on the Behavior, Reproduction, and Cortico Steroids of Male and Female Pigs," *Applied Animal Behavior Science* 15(1986):303–371; H. W. Gonyou et al., "Effects of Frequent Interactions with Humans on Growing Pigs," *Applied Animal Behavior Science* 16(1986):269–278.

68. National Pork Producers Council, *Swine Care Handbook,* pp. 14–15.

69. Temple Grandin, "Handling Problems Caused by Excitable Pigs," in *Proceedings of the 37th International Congress of Meat Science and Technology,* volume 1, September 1–6, 1991, Kulmbach, Germany. See also Stookey and Patience, "High Technology," p. 75.

70. Stanley Curtis, "Swine Welfare: Biology as the Basis" (paper presented at the annual meeting of the American Association of Swine Practitioners, 1990).

71. Grandin, "Handling Problems."

## Chapter 5. The Dairy Industry

1. M. F. Seabrook, "The Psychological Relationship between Dairy Cows and Dairy Cowmen and Its Implications for Animal Welfare," *Journal for the Study of Animal Problems* 1(1980):295–298.

2. See Roger Ewbank, "Stereotypies in Clinical Veterinary Practice," in *Proceedings of the First World Congress of Ethology and Applied Zootechnics* 1(1978):499 ff.

3. C. W. Arave and J. L. Albright, "Animal Welfare/Rights," work in progress, 1993; J. L. Albright and W. R. Stricklin, "Recent Developments in the Provision for Cattle Welfare," in C. J. C. Phillips (ed.), *New Techniques in Cattle Production* (London: Butterworth's, 1989), p. 149.

4. Mark Haake and Tim Waller, "Minimum Standards for Animal Care on Large Colorado Dairies" (paper for animal science class, Colorado State University, 1982).

5. J. L. Albright, "Our Industry Today," *Journal of Dairy Science* 66(1983):2208–2220.

6. J. L. Albright, "Dairy Animal Welfare: Current and Needed Research," *Journal of Dairy Science* 70(1987):2717.

7. Ibid., p. 2722.

8. J. L. Albright, "Review of Ruminant Behavior and Welfare Research," Journal paper no. 9575, Purdue University Agricultural Experiment Station (1983), p. 182.

9. Albright, "Dairy Animal Welfare," p. 2721.

10. J. H. B. Roy, *The Calf: Management and Feeding* (University Park: Pennsylvania State University Press, 1970).

11. Albright, "Our Industry Today," p. 2218.

12. Ibid.

13. Ronald Kilgour and Clive Dalton, *Livestock Behavior: A Practical Guide* (Boulder, Colo.: Westview, 1984), p. 13, citing H. H. Sambraus, "Humane Considerations in Calf Rearing," *Animal Regulation Studies* 3(1980):19–22.

14. Andrew Fraser and D. M. Broom, *Farm Animal Behaviour and Welfare,* 3d edition (London: Baillière Tindall, 1990), p. 353.

15. Albright, "Dairy Animal Welfare," p. 2722.

16. Ibid.

17. Fraser and Broom, *Farm Animal Behaviour,* p. 354.

18. M. W. Fox, *Farm Animals: Husbandry, Behavior, and Veterinary Practice* (Baltimore: University Park Press, 1984), p. 106.

19. Kilgour and Dalton, *Livestock Behavior,* p. 38.

20. Albright, "Dairy Animal Welfare," p. 2725.

21. Kilgour and Dalton, *Livestock Behavior,* p. 36.

22. *New York Times,* October 25, 1988.

23. Arave and Albright, "Animal Welfare/Rights," p. 4.

24. Kilgour and Dalton, *Livestock Behavior,* p. 32.

25. Personal communication, 1993.

26. Ronald Kilgour, "The Application of Animal Behavior and the Humane Care of Farm Animals," *Journal of Animal Science* 46(1978):1478–1486.

27. Fraser and Broom, *Farm Animal Behaviour,* p. 355.

28. F. J. Manson and J. D. Leaver, "Effect of Hoof Trimming and Protein Level on Lameness in Dairy Cows," *Animal Production* 42(1986):451; F. J. Manson and J. D. Leaver, "The Effect of Concentrate, Silage Ratio and of Hoof-trimming on Lameness in Dairy Cattle," *Animal Production* 49(1989):15–22.

29. *Management of Welfare of Farm Animals: The UFAW Handbook,* 3d edition (London: Baillière Tindall, 1988), p. 42.

30. Fraser and Broom, *Farm Animal Behavior,* p. 355.

31. *UFAW Handbook,* p. 42.

32. Kilgour, "Application of Animal Behaviour."

33. Haake and Waller, "Minimum Standards," p. 19.

34. Seabrook, "Psychological Relationship."

35. M. F. Seabrook, "Reactions of Dairy Cattle and Pigs to Humans," in R. Zayan and Robert Dantzer (eds.), *Social Stress in Domestic Animals* (Dordrecht: Kluwer, 1990), pp. 110–121.

36. Albright, "Dairy Animal Welfare."

37. Temple Grandin, "Livestock Handling Needs Improvement," *Animal Nutrition and Health* 40,7(1985):6.

38. *UFAW Handbook,* pp. 4–5.

39. Richard Bowen and Gordon Niswender, personal communication, 1993.

40. See detailed discussion in B. E. Rollin, *The Frankenstein Syndrome* , (New York: Cambridge University Press, 1995).

41. John Bocock, "Contented Cows—Concerned Consumers," in Jerome Martin (ed.), *High Technology and Animal Welfare* (Edmonton: University of Alberta, 1991), pp. 51–61.

42. Ibid., p. 55.

43. Ibid., p. 56.

44. Ibid., p. 57.

45. D. S. Kronfeld, "Management of Dairy Herds Treated with Bovine Somatotropin," *Journal of the American Veterinary Medical Association* 204,1(1994):116–130.

46. Preben Willeberg, "An International Perspective on Bovine Somatotropin and Clinical Mastitis," *Journal of the American Veterinary Medical Association,* 205,4(1994):538–540.

## Chapter 6. The Veal Industry

1. *The Animal Policy Report,* volume 7, number 1, April 1993 (Tufts University School of Veterinary Medicine Center for Animals and Public Policy), p. 5.

2. Andrew Fraser and D. M. Broom, *Farm Animal Behaviour and Welfare* (London: Baillière Tindall, 1988), p. 353.

3. John Webster, *Calf Husbandry, Health, and Welfare* (Boulder, Colo.: Westview, 1984).

4. John Webster, Claire Saville, and David Welchman, *Improved Husbandry Systems for Veal Calves* (Bristol: Animal Health Trust, Farm Animal Care Trust, 1986), p. 22.

5. T. H. Friend and G. R. Dellmeier, "Common Practices and Problems Related to Artificially Rearing Calves: An Ethological Analysis," *Applied Animal Behavior Science* 20(1988):47–62.

6. Ibid., p. 47.

7. Ibid., p. 49.

8. G. R. Dellmeier, T. H. Friend, and E. E. Gbur, "Comparison of Four Methods of Calf Confinement. II. Behavior," *Journal of Animal Science* 60(1985):1102–1109.

9. Fraser and Broom, *Farm Animal Behaviour*, p. 353.

10. J. G. de Wilt, *Behavior and Welfare of Veal Calves in Relation to Husbandry Systems* (Wageningen, Holland: IMAG, 1985).

11. Ibid., p. 353.

12. Friend and Dellmeier, "Common Practice," p. 50.

13. Ibid., p. 53.

14. Ibid., p. 57; M. W. Fox, *Farm Animals: Husbandry, Behavior, and Veterinary Practice* (Baltimore: University Park Press, 1984), Appendix B.

15. J. W. Mason, "A Re-evaluation of the Concept of 'Non-specificity' in Stress Theory," *Journal of Psychiatric Research* 8(1971):323–333; Jay Weiss, "Psychological Factors in Stress and Disease," *Scientific American* 226 (March 1972):101–113.

16. M. E. P. Seligman, *On Depression, Development, and Death* (San Francisco: W. H. Freeman, 1975).

17. Fraser and Broom, *Farm Animal Behaviour*, p. 354.

18. Webster et al., *Improved Husbandry Systems*, p. 17.

19. Fraser and Broom, *Farm Animal Behaviour*, p. 354.

20. Webster et al., *Improved Husbandry Systems*, p. 17.

21. Ibid., p. 21.

22. Fraser and Broom, *Farm Animal Behaviour*, p. 353.

23. Webster et al., *Improved Husbandry Systems*.

24. D. D. Johnson et al., "Effect of Calf Management on Carcass Characteristics and Palatability Traits of Veal Calves," *Journal of Dairy Science* 75(1992):2799–2804.

25. H. A. Agboola et al., "The Effects of Individual and Combined Feeding of High Monophosphate and α-tocopherol-supplemented Milk Replacer Diets and an Alternate Protein Diet on Muscle Color, Composition, and Cholesterol Content of Veal," *Journal of Animal Science* 68(1990):117 ff.

26. H. A. Agboola et al., "The Effects of a High Monosodium Phosphate and Alpha Tocopherol Supplemented Milk Replacer Diet on Veal Muscle Color and Composition," *Journal of Animal Science* 66(1988):1676–1685.

27. F. K. McKeith et al., "Enhancement of Lean Characteristics of Veal Carcasses by Electrical Stimulation," *Meat Science* 6(1982):65–69.

28. T. J. Seubert, "Loose Housing of Special Fed Veal Calves," *The Vealer*, July 1987, pp. 18–21.

29. Trevor Tomkins, "Loose Housing: Let's Get the Facts Straight!" *The Vealer*, December 1984, special section (emphasis added).

30. Ibid.

## Chapter 7. The Poultry Industry

1. Andrew Fraser and D. M. Broom, *Farm Animal Behaviour and Welfare*, 3d Edition (London: Baillière Tindall, 1990), p. 370.

2. M. E. Pennington, F. L. Platt, and C. G. Snyder, *Eggs* (Chicago: Progress Publications, 1933).

3. Ibid., p. 55.

4. Ibid., p. 244.

5. Ibid., pp. 248, 251.

6. Ruth Harrison, *Animal Machines* (London: Vincent Stuart, 1964).

7. Fraser and Broom, *Farm Animal Behaviour,* p. 370.

8. Ibid. See also J. P. Kruijt, "Autogeny of Social Behavior in Burmese Red Jungle Fowl (*Gallus gallus spadiceus*)," *Behavior* (1964), supplement 12.

9. Personal communication, 1989.

10. Pennington et al., *Eggs,* p. 284.

11. Jack Avens, personal communication, 1993.

12. Don Bell, "The Effects of Cage Density and Cage Shape," *California Poultry Letter,* Co-operative Extension, University of California, September 1988, p. 7.

13. Joy Mench, "The Welfare of Poultry in Modern Production Systems," in *CRC Critical Reviews in Poultry Biology,* volume 4, 1992, 107–128.

14. B. O. Hughes and I. J. H. Duncan. "The Influence of Strain and Environmental Factors upon Feather Picking and Cannibalism in Fowl," *British Poultry Science* 13(1972):525–547; I. J. H. Duncan and B. O. Hughes, "The Effect of Population Size and Density on Feather Picking." in *4th European Poultry Conference* (1973), pp. 473 ff.

15. Mench, *Welfare of Poultry,* p. 38.

16. Ibid, pp. 38–39.

17. Fraser and Broom, *Farm Animal Behaviour,* p. 383.

18. Mench, "Welfare of Poultry," p. 39.

19. Paul Siegel, personal communication, 1991.

20. M. W. Fox, *Farm Animals: Husbandry, Behavior, and Veterinary Practice* (Baltimore: University Park Press, 1984), p. 11.

21. D. G. M. Wood-Gush, *Elements of Ethology* (London: Chapman and Hall, 1983), passim.

22. Fraser and Broom, *Farm Animal Behaviour,* p. 374.

23. Ibid., p. 375.

24. Ibid.

25. Ibid.

26. H. B. Simonsen, "Ingestive Behavior and Wing-flapping in Assessing Welfare of Laying Hens," in D. Smidt (ed.), *Current Topics in Veterinary Medicine and Animal Science* 23 (The Hague: Martinus Nijhoff, 1983), pp. 89–95.

27. Fraser and Broom, *Farm Animal Behaviour,* p. 375.

28. Mench, "Welfare and Poultry," p. 18.

29. I. J. H. Duncan, "Frustration in the Fowl," in B. M. Freeman and R. F. Gordon (eds.), *Aspects of Poultry Behavior* (Edinburgh: British Poultry Science 1970), pp. 15–31.

30. D. G. M. Wood-Gush and A. B. Gilbert, "Observations on the Laying Behaviour of Hens in Battery Cages, *British Poultry Science* 10(1969):29.

31. Mench, "Welfare of Poultry," p. 19.

32. Ibid.

33. Ibid., pp. 16–17.

34. Ibid., p. 17.

35. Ronald Kilgour and Clive Dalton, *Livestock Behavior: A Practical Guide* (Boulder, Colo.: Westview, 1984), p. 192.

36. G. McBride et al., "The Social Organization and Behavior of the Feral Domestic Fowl," *Animal Behavior,* monograph 2(1969):127–181.

37. Kilgour and Dalton, *Livestock Behavior,* pp. 192–193.

38. B. O. Hughes, "Selection of Group Size by Individual Laying Hens," *British Poultry Science* 18(1977):9–18.

39. Mench, "Welfare of Poultry," p. 28.

40. Daniel Rosenberg, "Old World Primates," in B. E. Rollin and M. L. Kesel (eds.), *The Experimental Animal in Biomedical Research*, volume 2, (Boca Raton, Fla.: CRC Press, 1995).

41. See references in Fraser and Broom, *Farm Animal Behaviour*, p. 375.

42. Mench, "Welfare of Poultry," p. 29.

43. M. S. Dawkins and S. Hardie, "Space Needs of Laying Hens," *British Poultry Science*, 30(1989):413–416.

44. Mench, "Welfare of Poultry," p. 29.

45. Ibid., pp. 28–35.

46. I. J. H. Duncan and B. O. Hughes, "Free and Operant Feeding in Domestic Fowls," *Animal Behavior* 20(1972):775–777.

47. H. J. Blokhuis, "Feather Pecking in Poultry: Its Relation with Ground Pecking," *Applied Animal Behavior Science* 16(1986):63–67.

48. M. C. Appleby et al., "Behavior of Laying Hens in a Deep Litter House," *British Poultry Science* 30(1989):545–553.

49. Rosenberg, "Old World Primates."

50. *Management and Welfare of Farm Animals: The UFAW Handbook* (London: Baillière Tindall, 1988), p. 198.

51. Mench, "Welfare of Poultry," p. 20.

52. *UFAW Handbook*, p. 198.

53. Mench, "Welfare of Poultry," p. 21.

54. Fox, *Farm Animals*, p. 20.

55. *UFAW Handbook*, p. 198.

56. Fraser and Broom, *Farm Animal Behaviour*, p. 376.

57. Fox, *Farm Animals*, p. 14.

58. Fraser and Broom, *Farm Animal Behaviour*, p. 374.

59. George Seidel, personal communication, 1993.

60. See Mench, "Welfare of Poultry," p. 49 and references 197–200, 207, 258 therein; J. V. Craig and W. M. Muir, "Selection for Reduction of Beak-inflicted Injuries among Caged Hens, *Poultry Science* 72(1993):411–420.

61. See B. E. Rollin, *Animal Rights and Human Morality*, 2d edition (Buffalo, N.Y.: Prometheus Books, 1992).

62. Mench, "Welfare of Poultry, p. 49.

63. Fraser and Broom, *Farm Animal Behaviour*, p. 379.

64. Ibid., p. 378.

65. *UFAW Handbook*, p. 212.

66. David Sainsbury, *Farm Animal Welfare: Cattle, Pigs, and Poultry* (London: William Collins, 1986), p. 162.

67. Ibid., p. 165 (emphasis added).

68. Ibid.

69. Ibid., p. 166.

70. Ibid., p. 167.

71. Ibid., p. 164.

72. T. Tanaka and J. F. Hurnik, "Comparison of Behavior and Performance of Laying Hens Housed in Battery Cages and an Aviary," *Poultry Science* 71(1992):235–243 (emphasis added).

73. Ibid., p. 242.

74. M. C. Appleby et al., *Poultry Production Systems: Behavior, Management, and Welfare* (Wallingford, U.K.: CAB International, 1992).

75. Mench, "Welfare of Poultry," p. 3.

76. Fraser and Broom, *Farm Animal Behaviour*, p. 382.

77. I. J. H. Duncan, personal communication, 1993.

78. Fraser and Broom, *Farm Animal Behaviour,* p. 382.

79. I. J. H. Duncan, personal communication, 1993.

80. Ibid.

81. Ibid.

82. Fraser and Broom, *Farm Animal Behaviour,* p. 382.

83. Fox, *Farm Animals,* p. 6.

84. Fraser and Broom, *Farm Animal Behaviour,* p. 383.

85. Duncan, personal communication, 1993.

86. Mench, "Welfare of Poultry," p. 41.

87. I. J. H. Duncan et al., "Comparison of the Stressfulness of Harvesting Broiler Chickens by Machine and by Hand," *British Poultry Science* 27(1986):109.

88. Mench, "Welfare of Poultry," p. 42.

89. Ibid., p. 44.

90. Ibid., p. 45.

# Index